Int

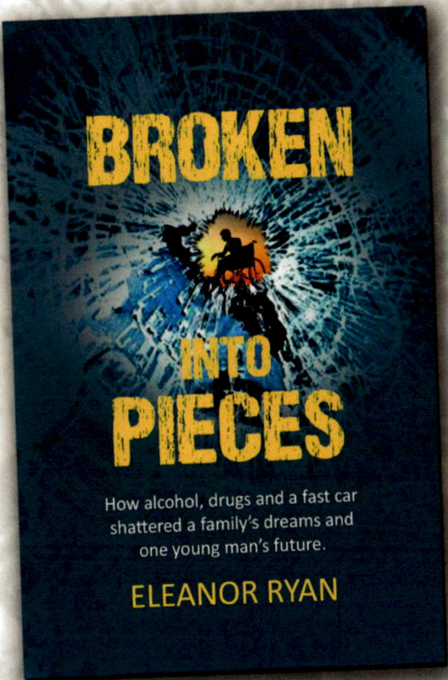

A New Book by

Eleanor Ryan

Raw, riveting and real, Broken into Pieces is a rollercoaster ride into the shattered lives of a teenager and his family. Following the toxic cocktail of youthful invincibility, a hot sports car and booze combined with a freak ice storm, Ron's car accident forever alters his future. This book is a fictionalized account of Ron Evans' true story.

Eleanor Ryan is an author and playwright whose short stories and poetry have been published in the annual Langley Writers Guild Chapbook, Canadian Stories, and other magazines. She has written and directed a number of award-winning one-act plays and is the author of the children's book, Dragons I Know. Broken into Pieces is Ryan's first novel.

The author lives with her husband, Phil, in Langley, B.C.

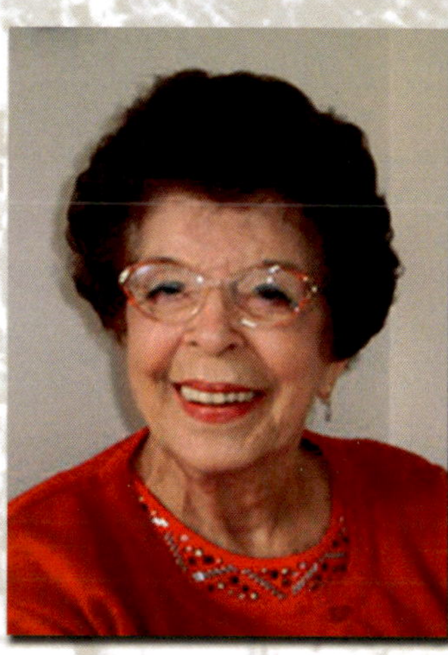

www.eleanorryan.ca

BROKEN into PIECES

Eleanor Ryan

BROKEN into PIECES

How alcohol, drugs and a fast car shattered a family's dreams and one young man's future.

Eleanor Ryan

RYAN PUBLICATIONS

RYAN PUBLICATIONS

While based on a true story of real experiences this book is a work of fiction. The information included is for general information only, and is not a substitute for the medical advice of a doctor or other health care professionals. The author is not responsible or liable for any diagnosis made by a user based on the content of this book. Names, places and circumstances have been changed to protect the privacy of the individuals involved.

Edited by Wendy Dewar Hughes
Interior Design and Cover Design:
Wendy Dewar Hughes, Summer Bay Press

RYAN PUBLICATIONS
20735 - 50B Avenue
Langley, B.C. V3A 7T9
E-mail: e_ryan@shaw.ca

ISBN: 978-0-9868775-7-5
Digital ISBN: 978-0-9868775-8-2

This book is dedicated to 'Ron' whose generosity and courage allowed me to tell his story, to convey his message, "If by telling my story, one kid is saved...then it will be worth it."

ACKNOWLEDGEMENTS

Per Ardua ad Astra

My heartfelt thanks go out to those angels of mercy and wisdom who presented themselves when needed most, as angels are wont to do. Through their generosity of spirit, expertise and compassion, they upheld and taught us, not by words alone, but by their fine example, to reach for the stars on our journey through adversity.

Members of the RCMP
Fire Rescue Emergency Services
Langley Memorial Hospital
Surrey Memorial Hospital
Vancouver General Hospital
G.F. Strong Rehabilitation Centre
Fraser Health Authority
Paraplegic Association
Acquired Brain Injury Association
Addictions Counsellors
ICBC Rehabilitation Services
Peter Methven, M.B., Ch. B., C.C.F.P.

My love and gratitude go out to my husband who waited with patience and often without dinner while I wrote "Broken into Pieces"'; to members of the Connolly, Celli, Ryan and Sprung families who continue in their loving support of 'Ron', I give my deepest love and appreciation.

Thanks also to those who inspired and encouraged me to keep on writing - my mentors, Ed Griffin, author/writing instructor, Wendy Dewar Hughes, author/book mentor, and members of the Langley Writers Guild.

ONE

"The West Coast can expect gale-force winds and rain turning to sleet later this evening. Road conditions may be hazardous, especially at the higher levels..."

The T.V. weatherman's voice droned on. As I cleared the kitchen table the sound of the television provided background accompaniment to the clatter of dishes and cutlery I dropped into the sink.

My husband, Jeff, called out from the adjacent family room, "Janice, do you have to make that racket? I'm trying to listen to the news."

The thermostat in the hallway registered seventy degrees but the house felt cold. I grabbed an old sweater from the hall closet and wrapped it around my shivering body. When I went back to the kitchen, I stopped for a moment and listened to the wind blowing through the maple trees in our back garden.

"Anybody seen my car keys?" Our eighteen-year-old son, Ron, shoelaces untied and cap on backwards, slouched into the family room and dug around under the sofa cushions until he found his keys. "How'd they land up there?" he asked, flipping them into his palm.

Jeff sat up, aimed his remote control at the television set and clicked it off. I heard him mumble something under his breath as he picked up the evening paper. With a grim look on his face he flipped it open.

Inspecting Ron's outfit, I asked, "Are you going out looking like that?"

"Ah, Mom, lay off, will you? I told you this afternoon I'm going over to Jason's to work on my car, remember? Anyway, all the guys wear stuff like this."

"Put on your winter jacket," I instructed. "It will be stormy tonight. The T.V. news forecast sleet later on so watch the road."

Ron groaned. "Just because I'm the youngest, you don't have to treat me like a little kid. You never talk to Kevin like that."

I pressed my lips together as I swished the soapy dishcloth over a dinner plate and looked out the window. An enormous cloud loomed in the evening sky. It had changed colour and shape from the fluffy, yellow-white look of the afternoon to an odd, grey-black layer that hovered over our house. It resembled a panther waiting to pounce. An uneasy shiver scampered down my spine.

"I'm not a little kid anymore, you know," Ron muttered as he shrugged on his leather jacket. Twirling his car keys around one finger, he headed out the door.

Jeff put down his newspaper and got up from his reclining chair. He brushed my cheek with a kiss. "I think I'll go to bed," he said. "I'm feeling a bit tired."

I watched him shuffle down the hallway then turned my attention back to the window. The clouds, dense and menacing, hung like evil spirits in the sky. From the window I saw Ron unlock the door of his new, red sports car and hop in. He whipped the seat belt across his chest and cranked the key in the ignition. The engine rumbled. Slamming the gear shift into reverse, he backed down the driveway and sped away. What am I going to do with that boy? I thought, shaking my head.

I turned away from the sink and looked down the hall. The bedroom door stood open a crack. Jeff's heart problem and a lingering infection had turned him into an old man almost overnight. I sighed and picked up another dish. Our plans for a long-awaited European vacation this year sat on a shelf gathering dust. The "good life" of fun and travel we had imagined for our retirement had taken a back seat to his health issues and black moods. I glanced out the window at the sky again as fat raindrops splashed against the window pane.

The rhythmic tap, tap of the rain thumped in rhythm to the pounding in my brain. I moved about the kitchen like an unseeing robot as I dried the dishes and stacked them in the cupboards. Scattered thoughts raced through my mind. This had not been one of my better days. At one moment I thought of Jeff and our future and in the next I brooded about Ron's sullen attitude of the past week. Tears welled up in my eyes. I wiped them away with the damp tea towel I still clutched in my hand then hung it on the handle of the stove.

The mellow brown leather of Jeff's chair looked inviting so I plugged the kettle in and threw a tea bag into a mug. Wisps of steam rose up from the bubbling kettle and as I bent over it they soothed my face. I poured the boiling water over the tea bag, wrapped both hands around the hot mug and sank into the cozy comfort of the easy chair.

Covering my legs with a well-worn lap robe, I curled up and savoured the taste and aroma of the steaming hot tea and as I began to feel more comfortable I picked up a novel I'd been reading. For some reason though, I couldn't shake off the feelings of anxiety that crawled like tiny bugs over my skin. I found myself reading the same page over and over until finally my eyelids grew heavy and I drifted into an uneasy after-dinner nap.

I awoke with a bang. A sudden gust of wind had caught the outside screen door and whipped it open, smashing it against the porch wall with such impact that the entire house rattled and jolted me out of my dream state. My book thudded to the floor. I untangled myself from the blanket wrapped around my legs and leapt to my feet. As I hurried to latch the flapping screen door, I braced myself against another, stronger gust of wind, so fierce and cold its blast stung my flesh.

Snapping the latch into place, I gripped my sweater tighter around my shoulders and looked up at the black and white dial of the kitchen clock. Ten-thirty. Sighing, I picked up the blanket and tossed it into the chair. I couldn't get Ron's curt statement, "I'm not a little kid anymore…," out of my mind, nor could I shake the familiar shadow of regret and guilt that followed me, mocking my every step, as though it was holding me to account. At least I could have given him a cheerful goodbye before he left the house, I thought.

I walked through the house checking for further wind damage then padded down the hall to our bedroom and peered in. I knew Jeff's loud snoring would grate on my nerves if I tried to sleep with him so I decided to lie down in the spare bedroom instead. Yet once snuggled down in the smaller bed, I tossed and turned in fitful sleep. During the night I woke up, rolled over, and squinted at the bedside clock. Like the warning light of a traffic signal, its yellow dial glowed through the darkness. Two o'clock and all is not well, it seemed to say. Filled with a sense of foreboding, I suddenly realized I hadn't heard Ron come home.

Crawling out of bed, I clutched my bathrobe around me and scurried down the hall to his room. He wasn't in his bed. With my emotional state swinging wildly between anxiety and annoyance, I sighed. Why hasn't he phoned? I seethed.

By now there was no point in going back to bed. I wouldn't sleep anyway so I plunked myself back down into Jeff's chair to wait for Ron to come home. A dull, heavy ache sat in the pit of my stomach and refused to go away. Where could he possibly be at this hour? Thinking back I recalled what he'd told me earlier that afternoon. "Uh, Mom, Jason called. He said it's okay to bring my car over tonight. His dad told him we could use his garage. I want to check my brakes."

Busy folding laundry, I had answered him vaguely, "Mm…all right."

Jason. I couldn't imagine his parents would

allow the boys to hang around until this hour of the morning. But then I thought, *maybe Jason's parents are away*. Or maybe Ron left their house to visit one of his girlfriends.

I glanced up at the kitchen clock once more. The stark black and white dial stared back at me as it tick-tocked three o'clock. I ran my hands through my hair then decided to risk the displeasure of Jason's parents at phoning his home this time of the night. A sleepy male voice I recognized as Jason's father, Gordon McDonald, answered. "Hullo. Who is this?"

"It's Janice Evans, Gordon. I'm sorry to wake you but Ron hasn't come home yet and I wondered if he was still at your place."

"Ron's not here, Janice. Good grief, it's after three! You mean he's still not home? Oh, wait a minute. Hold on and I'll wake up Jason." I could hear two voices mumbling in the background then Jason came on. "Hullo, Mrs. Evans?"

"Jason, Ron hasn't come home yet. I thought you might know where he's gone. He told me he'd be at your house. He left here before eight o'clock."

"Yeah, Ron had to leave early. One of the guys brought some booze with him. My Dad came out to the garage and caught us drinking. He got pretty mad and sent everybody home."

"I don't blame him for being angry. You and Ron are only eighteen, remember. "

"I know but we made sure Ron was okay before he got in the car. He didn't look drunk or anything, Mrs. Evans. There was this guy from Valleyview who didn't have a ride home and I think Ron gave him a lift. They left about eleven. He should have been home ages ago."

I asked for the other fellow's name and phone number. "Gee, I'm sorry. I didn't get his name. He just turned up. He's a tall, skinny guy, older than us; maybe twenty. He had sort of sandy hair and a thin moustache but I can't tell you any more than that."

"It's all right, Jason. Go back to bed. I'll call you when I hear from Ron."

I put the phone down. Terror seized every inch of my body as once again my eyes focused on the dial of the kitchen clock. Four o'clock, it taunted, its second hand racing in time to the thumping of my heart. It's four o'clock and still no call. This isn't like Ron. He'd phone home if he could. I felt gripped with the certainty that something had happened; something very bad.

Jeff stumbled out of the bedroom. "Do you know what time it is?" he growled. "What the hell's going on?"

"Ron's not home yet, Jeff. It's after four. I'm calling the police."

Jeff's face turned grey. He dropped down into his chair as his hand reached for his nitro spray, "Jan...Jan."

I snatched the container from his hand and sprayed the medication directly into his open mouth. Almost immediately, his colour returned. He uttered an oath. "That damned car! I told you we shouldn't have let him buy a sports car. The motor is too powerful for a young kid to handle."

"Don't start, Jeff. Blaming me won't solve anything. I'm going to make that call."

The portable phone had disappeared. I'd put it down somewhere after talking to the McDonalds but couldn't remember where. Jeff turned and twisted in his chair then reached behind his back and pulled out the wayward phone. I grabbed it from his hand and dialled.

"Ogden Police, Constable Johanson."

"This is Janice Evans, Constable. I'm calling to report my son missing."

"Please spell your last name, ma'am."

"E-v-a-n-s, Janice Evans. My son's name is Ronald Evans. He's..."

"R-o-n-a-l-d E-v-a-ns? His age, ma'am?"

"That's right. He's eighteen. He left his friend's house last night about eleven o'clock with another person and..."

"Eighteen, and he's been missing for how

long?"

I took a quick breath and all my anxiety began to pour out of me.

"Mrs. Evans, I'll ask you to stop right there. As I understand it, your son left his friend's place about eleven last night. It's four-thirty a.m. now. That's five and a half hours."

"But you don't understand. He wouldn't stay out this late without phoning home."

"I'll take a description of your son and his vehicle, and a description of his passenger. There's little else I can do at this time. For the record, please give me your full name again as well as your street address and telephone number."

The officer's endless questions annoyed me. His manner seemed understanding enough but at that moment I wanted to jump through the phone and shake him. Didn't he realize that, although Ron's well-being might not be a high police priority, as his mother, it had to be mine?

"Jeff! What's Ron's license plate number?"

Jeff, who always remembered such details, shouted across the room, "It's not a number. Have you forgotten? We bought him a special license plate for his birthday. It's "BAD BOY"." BAD BOY. At the time I had thought Ron's chosen name for his license plate bordered on the ridiculous but he'd insisted on having that name plate for his birthday present.

After I turned back to the phone and gave the officer that special piece of information, he advised, "If you don't hear from him within the next hour or two, you might want to give Ogden Hospital a call, ma'am."

"What did he say?" asked Jeff after I hung up. I repeated the officer's advice.

I imagined Ron lying injured somewhere, unable to call home, and felt sick. Jeff's expression turned from irritation to concern. He got up and began to make a pot of coffee. "We'll need some strong coffee to get us through the rest of the night, Jan."

I moved over to stand beside him and put my head down on his shoulder.

"There, there, honey," he said, patting my head. "It'll be okay. Boys of his age, you know how they are. I'll bet he's fast asleep at some girl's house."

If that turns out to be true, I thought, I will never again lecture Ron about his sex life.

"Are you going to be okay?' Jeff asked.

"I'll be fine," I lied, punching the number of Ogden hospital into the phone dial. The response from our small local hospital was the same as from the police. They hadn't admitted anyone during the night who fit Ron's description.

When we heard the bedside clock ring its six o'clock alarm Jeff and I both looked up at the kitchen clock. Jeff rushed into the bedroom to silence the alarm's incessant ringing as I looked up once more at the bare face of the kitchen clock. A children's rhyme rattled through my thoughts. Sixty-six, clickety click, sixty-six, the devil plays tricks.

Jeff came back, took one look into my staring eyes, grabbed my arms from behind and forced me to sit down at the kitchen table. I couldn't move, my gaze fixed upon the hypnotic face of that damned clock. Sixty-six, clickety-click, sixty-six, the devil plays tricks, the voice in my head taunted.

"Drink this Jan. It'll help you focus," Jeff said, handing me a cup of black coffee. "It's been a rough night. You've done all you can for now."

"Could you find me a cigarette?" I pleaded. "I could do with a smoke about now." I had been trying to quit but right now I needed a smoke.

"Sure. I think I saw some in the cupboard." He squeezed my shoulder. "It's all right. You can quit smoking another day."

A few drags from the cigarette made me dizzy but the hit of nicotine along with Jeff's potent coffee brought me out of my trance. I began to think straight again. Jeff's dark mood seemed to have lifted. Maybe being forced to think about something other than his own illness would do him some good, I thought then immediately regretted my meanness.

At seven o'clock I answered a call from the police. Grasping the edge of the kitchen counter, I attempted to absorb the constable's message. "We received a fax from the Valleyview police, Mrs. Evans. They responded to a single vehicle accident in their area about one o'clock this morning."

"But Ron…?" I interrupted the constable.

"Mrs. Evans, please. We're not certain your son is involved. The victims are unidentified at this point. All I can tell you is the driver and his passenger were taken by ambulance to Valleyview Memorial."

Victims. The word seemed so distant, impersonal. "You might want to call Valleyview Emergency. They should be able to tell you more."

The knuckles of my hand turned white as I gripped the telephone. Looking across the room at Jeff, I began to weep.

"What is it, Jan?" He wrenched the phone from my hand. "Here, let me take it."

Clutching the back of a kitchen chair, I listened to Jeff's end of the conversation. His shoulders slumped. The telephone fell onto its cradle with a clatter as it dropped from his shaky hand. He turned stricken eyes to me. "Do you want to call Valleyview Hospital or should I?"

"I will. Their Emergency Department will know more about the people they admitted than the Ogden Police. Oh, the number. Jeff, do you have the number?" I shrieked.

"Yeah, yeah, calm down," he said, handing me a piece of notepaper he'd scribbled on while talking to the police.

The town of Valleyview bordered on our municipality of Ogden. I recalled Jason had told me that Ron's passenger lived in Valleyview. Everything began to fit. I glanced down at the paper Jeff handed me. With fingers trembling, I tapped the number into the phone pad.

"Valleyview Emergency," said a voice on the other end.

My name is Janice Evans. I'd like some information about a patient…"

"One moment please. I'll transfer you to the ward nurse."

After a long wait, a nurse picked up the extension. "Mrs. Evans?"

"Yes, Janice Evans. The Ogden Police told

me I should call you to enquire about two people who'd been injured in a motor vehicle accident this morning. We were told they'd been taken to Valleyview Memorial. My son didn't arrive home last night…"

"I understand, Mrs. Evans. Wait a moment. I'll check our files. Yes, two accident victims, both young males, were brought into our emergency ward early this morning. One has been released with no obvious injuries. The other victim however, had to be transferred to Drydon General because of the serious nature of his injuries. I'd advise you to contact Drydon Emergency for further information."

"But, I…"

"I'm sorry. That's the only information I have on file."

"Is it Ron?" Jeff hovered over me, his brow furrowed with concern.

"They don't know for sure." I put the phone down. "The nurse told me one person has been released with no injuries. But the other one is more seriously hurt and had to be transferred to Drydon General."

"Drydon? That's forty miles away. I guess if he's seriously hurt, the bigger hospital has specialists." He hesitated then added, "At least one of them is okay. Maybe it's Ron. He could be all right, Jan."

"If Ron could contact us, he would. I'm calling Drydon Emergency. I can't stand not knowing. Injured or not Jeff, we have to find him."

I looked past my husband and out the window. Weak sunlight filtered through the clouds as they drifted past on their journey east. The driving, icy rain and strong winds of the night before had subsided but I had a feeling we hadn't seen the last of the storm.

TWO

My heart pounded so hard I thought it might leap out of my chest. I gasped in some air and spoke. "My name is Janice Evans," I said when the voice had answered at Drydon Emergency. "The Valleyview Emergency nurse advised me to call you about a young man injured in a car accident who was transferred to Drydon this morning. My son…"

The woman cut me off. "One moment please. I'll connect you to the ward supervisor."

The phone clicked over to some recorded music making me feel even more on edge. Another click, a murmuring of voices, then at last, "Mrs. Evans? This is Evelyn Burns, Ward Supervisor."

"Yes. My son has been missing for hours and Valleyview Memorial told us…"

My practiced speech was interrupted as the nurse's voice cut in. "Mrs. Evans, we do have an unknown male in our emergency ward. If there's a possibility he's your son, we'd advise you to come to Drydon Emergency as soon as possible."

"But his I.D, have you looked in his pockets…?"

"I'm sorry. I can't give you specific information over the telephone. You'll need to come to the hospital in person if you believe you can identify our patient."

The phone fell from my limp hand and landed on the table. Jeff picked it up and placed it back on its cradle. "Please Jan. You've got to sit down."

"No. I have to drive into Drydon. The nurse wants me to come in and see if I can identify their patient. Dear God, Jeff, he must be unconscious or she wouldn't have said that."

Jeff paced across the tile floor of the kitchen. "Don't let your imagination run wild just yet. They don't know who he is for sure. It could be someone else. Lots of people are involved in accidents all around Drydon over the weekend."

I wasn't paying attention. I needed to run to my car, get on the highway and drive. I had to find Ron.

Jeff stopped his pacing and blurted out, "I'll get dressed. We'll both go."

"No, it would be better if you stayed here," I stated in a feeble attempt to take control of an otherwise out-of-control situation. "You're still not well enough to handle the stress. Someone has to stay by the phone in case there's any news. You get hold of George and ask him to come over. I'll feel better if someone stays here with you." George, Jeff's good buddy of many years, would be the ideal person to keep him company.

My brain switched into automatic mode as I barked out more orders to Jeff about writing everything down. Flying from kitchen to bathroom to bedroom then back to the kitchen again, I dressed, grabbed my purse and keys, and ran out to the car. On the way, I passed George, gave him a quick wave and leapt into the driver's seat. Twisting the key in the ignition I gave the gearshift a mighty yank, backed out of the carport and headed for the highway. Fasten your seat belt, girl, I told myself. You're in for a crazy ride.

I drove to Drydon in a daze. The speedometer registered sixty miles per hour but it seemed the car floated above the early morning fog as it moved, like an undulating snake along the winding highway. I felt imprisoned in its misty cocoon and my jailer's name was Fear.

By the time I reached the exit to Drydon, the fog had lifted. The sky cleared and I sped like a fiend through the narrow, tree-lined streets of the city. At Main Street I spied the familiar outline of the city's General Hospital. Swinging into the nearest parking spot, I flung open the car door and ran to get a ticket from the meter which I found a good half block away. I swiped my credit card and grabbed my ticket then raced back to the car, threw the ticket on the dashboard and ran toward the entrance.

The Emergency sign shone blood red. Emergency, emergency, it signalled in the early morning light. I couldn't stop thinking about Ron. My anxiety level increased by the second as I hurled myself through the automatic doors. The building foyer looked empty except for a maintenance worker slopping the floor with murky water from his bucket. I skidded to a stop. As he mopped his way in slow motion down the long corridor, the faded colour of his blue overalls merged with the hospital-green of the walls. Waves of ice-cold dread washed over me like the tide over an arctic shore.

A high-domed ceiling spanned the entire space. I wanted to shout but imagined that my voice would echo through the room like so much white noise, heard yet unintelligible and all my burning questions would hang unanswered in the void. On the other side of the lobby I spotted the reception area. Breathless, I approached a young nurse seated behind the desk. She looked up.

"Yes?"

"I'm Janice Evans. I called earlier about my son..."

"Ah, yes, Mrs. Evans." She glanced down at the mustard-brown file in front of her. "Would you come with me, please?" The slight, dark young woman led me into a small anteroom, empty except for a wall cupboard, a square table with metal legs and two folding chairs. "Please sit down," she said as she moved to the cupboard, removed a brown paper bundle and placed it on the table in front of me.

Her green scrubs blended in with the green, flaking paint of the walls. Hospital odours swirled about me and seemed like they were seeping through the pores of my skin. I felt sick. To add to the mix, spinning around in my throbbing head rang a familiar children's song, something about being green.

Seated at the table, I shivered in the thin mismatched outfit I had thrown on in my mad dash from the house. How long has it been, I wondered, since my maternal antenna rose in alarm? Heavy steel doors marked, "No Entrance" swung open on stout hinges and closed again with a metallic rasp. The sound grated upon my nerves, now raw from anxiety and lack of sleep.

The nurse glanced at me from under her dark bangs and with gloved hands opened the paper bundle. "This is the clothing removed from our patient. I'd like you to look at it and tell me if there is anything you recognize." On the table sat a pile of blood-soaked clothing, a pair of jeans, and a tee shirt, twisted and torn. On top of the pile lay a single, untied running shoe.

"No. Not my son's," I managed to croak. "Not Ron's," I insisted, turning my gaze away from the horrible sight. The clothes could belong to Ron's passenger, I thought, no, I hoped. But I felt ashamed as soon as the selfish notion entered my mind. That boy had a mother, too.

"Just a moment," the nurse murmured. She turned around as her older colleague padded into the room on cushioned nurse feet. "If you feel up to it, Mrs. Evans, we'd like you to come with us and see the patient."

A voice in my head screamed. But there's been a mistake. Where is the other boy's mother? Why am I the chosen one?

With a nurse on each side, the two women led me into an adjoining room where a limp figure lay on a raised bed, silent and unmoving. Beneath the bed, a chrome-clad X-frame, firm and fixed, stood its ground.

Why have they brought me to this hellish place? The person lying in front of me, so still, cannot be my son. No! Ron is good-looking and full of life. Everyone says so. No one could mistake his features, so unlike those of this poor unknown soul who lies here with his head so blue and swollen; so bloody and battered. No! No! This is not Ron, not this "victim".

Rigid, I strained against the nurses' firm hold as they continued to press, to guide my steps closer to the figure on the bed. I noticed a tangled maze of plastic tubes and wires attached to his body. They snaked across the bed sheet and up into a computerized black metal box. It sat there, beeping and flashing in response to whatever life remained in this broken body.

I began to shake uncontrollably.

The nurses continued to tug at my arms, as they led me closer to the side of the bed. My legs turned to water. I fell back into their waiting arms as I recognized beneath the layers of blood and dirt, my son's matted brown curls.

I don't remember how I got there but the next thing I knew I found myself in another room, seated on a drab brown and yellow striped armchair. A cup of tea sat on a small table beside me. The same young nurse I'd first met stood behind me. She covered my quivering shoulders with a warm blanket.

"There. Is that a little better, Mrs. Evans?" she asked as she placed my purse on the table.

I wanted to thank her but my mouth refused to form the words. My eyes darted around the rest of the room. Magazines waiting in precise rows for someone to pick them up languished unread on the coffee table. Across from the table another chair and a small sofa, upholstered in the same sickening brown and yellow stripes, sat as if in expectation of their next occupants. A black metal table off by itself in a corner held a telephone, telephone book, and an economy-size box of tissues.

Jeff. I must call Jeff, I thought, panic rising. But as I reached for the telephone it seemed to change form, to collapse in on itself and melt into the black table top.

The nurse sat on the arm of the chair. She held my hand as a tall, well-built man in blue scrubs, wearing a flowered print bonnet on his head, entered the room. He sat down in the chair opposite mine. My eyes watered from the chemical odour that wafted into the room with him.

"Mrs. Evans? Do you have any family with you in Drydon?

"No. My husband…" I stammered. I tried

to speak but my mind and tongue wouldn't cooperate. I felt the nurse squeezing my hand. I held on to her as a drowning sailor would to a life preserver.

"Evans? Your son's name is Ronald Evans?

I stared into his brown eyes, unable to communicate with the man.

"Mrs. Evans, your son has been involved in a motor vehicle accident. He is comatose at this time. I am sorry. He has sustained serious head and spinal injuries."

I didn't want to listen but nodded automatically in response to his voice. My resentment toward him grew as he continued to convey his awful message. I bit my lip, determined not to comprehend. As if imprisoned in a bad dream, I tried to prevent his dreadful news from breaking through the barrier my mind had thrown up in its defence. I caught bits and pieces of words, phrases, medical jargon.

"Spinal cord severed; paralyzed; closed head injury; unresponsive." His offer of help echoed throughout the room. "…anyone you would like me to call? The chaplain will come in to see you."

But his words had nothing to do with my burning need to wake up from this living nightmare. I felt the nurse's arms tighten around my shoulders. A strangled wail filled the tiny room. I knew the voice was mine but I failed to quiet its disconsolate lament. With every inch of my body immobilized I had somehow become the paralyzed, unresponsive one.

Then it was like something exploded in my brain. I opened my eyes to see an impenetrable curtain of red; a thick wall of fury and anguish. The wall then became black and then, nothing.

I had fainted.

THREE

The door to the waiting room swung open. I struggled to my feet as Jeff and George entered the room. Jeff ran to me, pulled me into his arms and kissed my wet cheeks.

"I've been to see him. The nurse from emergency called to tell me. Oh, God, Jan. Oh, dear God, our poor boy," he moaned, his entire body shaking with grief. We clung to each other, unable to say or do anything to ease our pain.

George leaned against the door frame, his iron-grey head bowed. "I'll go down and put some more money in the meter." His husky voice cracked with emotion. "You two take all the time you need. I'll grab a paper and sit in the coffee shop for a while. Call my cell when you need me, Jeff."

Jeff lifted his head and turned, his movements slow and heavy. "Thanks, George. We're okay for now." He slid an arm around my back and led me over to the sofa. Together, we sank down into its soft cushions and wept.

I must have slept because I woke up with a blanket and pillow bunched around me in an untidy heap at one end of the couch. Pale winter sun filtered through beige draperies and the striped upholstery had taken on a golden hue. Jeff lay sprawled at the other end of the couch, his mouth open. A soft snore escaped his dry lips. His left hand gripped my ankle.

I sat up, pushed my fingers through my hair and untangled my legs from the blanket. The door opened and a chubby middle-aged nurse strode into the room.

"Mr. and Mrs. Evans?" Her voice had a girlish tone that belied her age.

Jeff sat up, rubbed his reddened eyes and tugged his shirt down over his belly.

"Your son has been transferred to the Intensive Care Unit. You may go and sit with him now. Our neurologist, Doctor Fieldman, will meet you there in about ten minutes." She gathered up the blanket and pillow I had tossed aside and left the room.

Jeff's hand shook. He dug around in his jacket pocket, took out his pill box and without any water, tossed a couple of tablets down his throat.

"Are you sure you're up to this, Jeff?"

"Yeah, I'll be alright," he said, shoving the box back into his pocket. "I'd like to hear what this Doctor Fieldman has to say. I promise I'll call George and go straight home after that.

You need to get some rest yourself," he added, eyeing my stained, rumpled clothing.

"Oh, no!" I cried, clutching at his sleeve. I realized I hadn't given a single thought to our eldest son since before the accident. "Have you called Kevin?"

"I called. Don't worry. He's flying in later today." He stood up and stuffed his shirt tail into his waistband.

Everything will be better when Kevin is here, I thought. The family rock, Ron's big brother always seemed to know what to do in an emergency. I stood up and adjusted my clothing and mentally made out my 'things-to-do-next' list. Intensive Care Unit, sit with Ron, meet the neurologist, go to the bathroom, Intensive Care Unit, see Ron, neurologist... My head felt like it spun.

Jeff dragged me behind him through the maze of hospital corridors, tapping his foot as we waited for the elevator. I tried to pay attention to landmarks along the way. I had a notion that if I did then later I'd be able to backtrack to the hospital entrance and parking lot by myself. In the end I knew I wouldn't be able to recall one twist or turn of a hallway or distinguish one floor from another. I had more important things on my mind.

When we reached the I.C.U. we were

stopped by a male nurse who escorted us to a cramped waiting area. This one was different from those on the first floor. I felt the room closing in on me. Metal chairs lined up like soldiers leaned against the green walls of the windowless room. There were two telephones on the wall, one for calling outside the hospital and the other to ring for entrance into the I.C.U. Jeff started to read the page of directions stapled beside the last one. He turned toward me, "We have to call the nursing station for admittance," he informed me. "Visitors are restricted to those on the authorized visitors list."

He dialled through to the nursing station. "This is Jeff Evans, Ronald Evans' father. My wife and I would like to see our son. We have an appointment with Doctor Fieldman."

A loud buzzer sounded and the inner door lock clicked open. Jeff and I walked into a new and different ward. I sensed immediately the serious, down-to-business tone of the place. Ron's bed had been placed in the cubicle nearest to the nursing station.

Holding hands, we checked in at the station and were allowed to proceed. As we came close to his cubicle, a petite Asian nurse bustled about arranging something near the foot of Ron's bed. She looked up to greet us.

Her shining, dark eyes crinkled as she smiled. "Mr. and Mrs. Evans? My name's Grace. I'm Ronald's nurse. I'll be caring for him until the end of my shift and then another nurse will take over. He won't be left alone at any time." She moved to the head of the bed and looked at something on his intravenous line.

I tried to return her smile but could only manage some inane response. My face felt frozen, immobilized like the rest of my body. Why can't I get control of myself? I despaired. Jeff pulled my hand from his and I realized that I had dug my fingernails with such ferocity into his palm that they had drawn blood. I moved to the bedside and reached over to stroke Ron's swollen head. As I bent down to put my face against his I breathed in the warmth of his skin. The familiar smell of his body rose to envelop me and I became lost in a one-way embrace with my unconscious boy.

Jeff lifted me to my feet. We stood side-by-side, neither one of us attempting to break away from the side of the bed. My whole being ached at the sight of Ron's blood-soaked, shoulder-length hair as it lay spread out upon the white sheet, framing his bruised and battered head.

Jeff's thin body began to tremble. "Jan, I'm

sorry. I'll have to call George to drive me home after all. Will you be okay to meet the doctor by yourself?"

"You don't look well at all," I said. Feigning confidence I didn't feel, I continued, "You go straight home with George. Are you having chest pains?"

Jeff straightened up. "No. I feel weak, that's all."

"Then call George and go down to meet him now. Don't worry about me. Kevin should be here soon." I took note of his unsteady gait as he shuffled out of the ward.

Grace got up to close the curtains around the bed. Trapped within the claustrophobic cubicle, I felt overwhelmed by a deep sense of foreboding. After a moment, one corner of the curtain lifted and the doctor I'd been waiting to see stepped in. He extended a chubby hand, "Mrs. Evans, I'm Doctor Fieldman."

The first thing I noticed was his shoes. They were bright yellow; as yellow as buttercups on a morning in May. My startled gaze rose upward to take in his rotund shape. It didn't take long because his legs were so short. The diamond pattern of his black and yellow tie almost blinded me. Black-rimmed spectacles and a shiny blue suit completed this vision of sartorial splendour. When I looked into his eyes, I caught a reassuring glimpse of keen intelligence and compassion.

Without waiting for me to reply to his introduction he began, "The boy has sustained a closed head injury as well as a complicated spinal injury. We are most concerned about the hematoma and swelling in the brain. He remains comatose and we may have to consider brain surgery if the swelling doesn't go down. I've conferred with Doctor Newcomb, our spinal surgeon. While we agree he needs immediate surgery on his spine we think it best to postpone it for a few days to monitor the swelling in his brain."

Before he could go on, I interrupted him. Blubbering, I choked out, "But his legs…"

Doctor Fieldman continued, "Mrs. Evans, an appointment with the spinal surgeon will be made for you soon. As I said, I have conferred with Doctor Newcomb. Your son's spinal cord was severed in the accident. I'm so sorry. He won't walk again."

"But…you said…surgery," I sobbed.

"Yes. He needs surgery to stabilize the spine, to mend the damaged vertebrae. But the spinal cord itself can't be repaired."

"His legs…," I repeated, thinking about the skiing holiday he'd planned with his buddies.

"Our main concern right now is the head

injury. If there is no improvement, then spinal surgery will pose a challenge. We'll wait a few days and then make a decision."

Doctor Fieldman gripped my shoulder with a firm hand, "Goodbye Mrs. Evans. Try to get some rest. You've had a great shock. It will be some time before we can determine our next course of action." With that the doctor turned and made a rapid exit from the unit.

"Would you like a cup of tea?" The concern in Grace's voice brought me out of my stupor. "There's a kettle in the waiting room. You go ahead. I'll take good care of him," she said as she placed her hand on my shoulder and turned me around to face the exit. A cup of tea? What good would that do? What I needed was a good stiff drink right about now! I willed my wobbly legs to carry me back to the waiting room.

"Mom!" a familiar voice called as I opened the door. There, across the room, his arms outstretched, stood my son Kevin. Kevin had always reminded me of a dark nut chocolate with a delicious cream centre because his outer shell usually appeared a little rough but at his core there lay a sweet and tender soul. I breathed a long sigh and leaned my head against his broad chest. As his heartbeat echoed mine I drew comfort and strength from his presence.

"Dad filled me in. I'm going in to see Ron now. Afterward I'll drive you straight home. What you need is a hot bath and a good sleep. We've got a long road ahead of us, Mom. It's doubtful Dad will cope well. You know I'll do whatever I can to help but you have to stay strong. You have to take care of yourself or you won't be able to help Ron."

As I listened to Kevin's reasonable argument I made an effort to pull myself together. While he visited his brother, I passed the time making tea in the empty waiting room. I sat down on one of the metal chairs, sipped my tea, and for the first time since Ron's accident, took Kevin's advice and tried to relax.

FOUR

I stepped into the hot bath and breathed in the luxurious perfume of bath oil. As I lowered myself into the steaming water, bath bubbles surrounded my body and rose up to pop under my nose.

Kevin had been right, of course. I did need to remove myself from the stress of the past two days. I'll drive into the hospital tomorrow bright and early, I thought, as my eyelids drooped with exhaustion and the soothing warmth of the bath.

The next morning didn't begin as bright and early as I'd planned. I had slept soundly until nine o'clock but finally felt ready to face the day.

"I wrote a phone message down for you," Jeff said as he poured coffee into my cup. "They called from Doctor Newcomb's office with an appointment for this afternoon."

In the couple of days that had passed since the accident, Jeff and I agreed I would look after most of the day-to-day hospital duties while he and Kevin held down the fort at home. Since Kevin could only arrange for a two-week absence from work, in between their hospital visits he and Jeff planned to look after the house together. Laundry had piled up and grocery shopping had to be done. It seemed like a good plan for the next two weeks. Long-term arrangements could wait until later.

After breakfast, dressed and freshly made-up, I grabbed my purse and keys, kissed my family goodbye and scrambled into the car. I took a deep breath and tried to prepare myself for the long drive into the big city.

If only I could control my wild imaginings, I can get through this, I thought as I put the car in gear and steered toward the highway. I couldn't erase the vision of Ron in a coma lying as still as death in a hospital bed. Never could I have imagined that scene. I wondered, as I drove the winding highway, if the time would ever come when I could accept the gravity, the reality, of it all.

The car purred along as if it could navigate the route without any help from me until I realized with a jolt that I had swerved to the left and crossed the line. Jerking the car back into my own lane I was seized with a giggling fit of hysteria. I didn't have control over anything, not even the damned car, I thought as tears streamed down my cheeks.

I pulled over onto the next wide area at the

side of the road. I had to calm down. I must attend to my driving or one of these trips into Drydon would end in another catastrophe. Wives, mothers, are supposed to handle whatever comes their way. That's what you'd like to think, taunted the nagging little voice in my head. I failed to recognize that I had become a master of self-deception. If I lost control, my whole world would come tumbling down around my ears. I had never felt so alone in all my life.

Once I arrived at the hospital, I found the unit, this time without any problem, and went in to visit Ron. One couldn't exactly call it a visit because Ron didn't take part but I kept myself occupied. I found a washcloth and filled a basin with warm water. Swallowing back tears, I dipped the cloth into the soapy water and washed his hands and his bruised, swollen face. He hadn't moved at all so the bed didn't need much tidying but I needed to be doing something, anything.

The same nurse I had met on our first day came in. As she checked the monitors she explained her concern about pressure sores appearing on Ron's body. "They can occur when the body is immobile and constant pressure is put upon the skin," she told me. "That can cause the skin to break down. A pressure sore can ulcerate in a very short time so the immobile patient's position must be changed often." Another nurse came in to help as it took two nurses to move him. With one on either side, they performed what they called a log-roll maneuver to turn him on his other side.

"You haven't had any lunch yet, Mrs. Evans," the nurse reminded me after I had been there some time. "Perhaps you should take a break."

I looked up at the ward clock that ticked off the minutes until my two o'clock appointment with Doctor Newcomb. His office was in another building so I grabbed a coffee and donut on my way and arrived for my appointment just in time.

The surgeon popped his head into the waiting room and motioned me to follow him. When I walked behind him into his office I noticed his sturdy build. He looked extremely fit. My eyes glanced down at his large hands that ended in fine long fingers, well-suited to his profession, I imagined.

"We haven't met, Mrs. Evans. I'm Doctor Newcomb. I'll be performing your son's spinal surgery. Please take a seat," he said, indicating a green leather tub chair in front of his desk.

He sat down, opened a yellow file folder and furrowed his brow. "Ron needs immediate spinal surgery. I've discussed this with Doctor Fieldman and we've decided not to wait any longer. His surgery is booked for today at six p.m."

"Today? So soon? I'll have to call my husband. He'll..."

"Yes, of course. I want you both to understand the risks involved considering his brain injury...the anaesthesia..."

Once again I was taken back to the night of the accident in that awful place, listening to a litany of things that could go wrong. And I heard, not the surgeon's exact words, but my own crazy, interpretation of them. I listened to the phrases; bits and pieces of medical jargon. I wanted to run out of his office but I sat frozen to the chair while my head nodded up and down like a bobble-head figure.

He paused, his fine features drawn with concern, and leaned over the desk and wrapped his surgeon's hands around mine. He made me a promise. "We'll do our utmost for your son, Mrs. Evans," he said. When I looked into Doctor Newcomb's sincere blue eyes, I felt almost certain I could trust him with Ron's life.

I had no memory of returning from the surgeon's office to the I.C.U. waiting room. Jeff and Kevin appeared out of nowhere. I supposed the doctor had had his nurse call them about Ron's impending surgery.

Jeff held an official-looking form in his hand. His voice trembled, "We have to give them permission to perform Ron's surgery."

"Yes, the doctor explained it to me. He told me the operation is risky but it has to be done." I held my hand out to Jeff so he could give me the paper. "I'll sign it first and you can put your signature below mine."

"Okay," he agreed, and passed the form to me as if it was too hot for his hand.

I took a pen from my purse and before I had time to think about it signed the form. I felt like I had just signed Ron's death warrant.

Kevin took the paper out of my hand and gave it to his father. "Okay, Dad, your turn."

Sucking in his breath Jeff wrote his signature on the bottom of the form and gave it to the nurse who added it to her growing file.

"'Round and 'round I go, down and down I go, in a spin…'". The song lyrics ran over and over in my mind. They described my emotions as I watched, along with my husband and Kevin, the green-suited O.R. staff as they bundled Ron in sheets and placed him gently on their gurney. The clock on the wall indicated the approaching event. Five o'clock.

We followed the wheeled gurney into the

elevator which rose to the surgical floor. When we exited the elevator Kevin pointed out the long hallway leading to the operating theatre. I felt cold and drew closer to Jeff. The three of us stood there and waited as the staff rolled Ron's gurney out of elevator after us.

One by one we bent over to touch him; to say good-by in case this might be our last chance then they whisked him away to the operating room. We stayed rooted to the hall floor until the gurney disappeared through the swinging doors of the O.R.

A few minutes later, Ron's surgeon and his assistant approached in their green scrubs. Doctor Newcomb gave us a reassuring smile. "Ron's tests look fine so far and his anesthesiologist is the best. He's in good hands, folks. It will be a lengthy surgery but we'll look after him."

Kevin walked beside Jeff and me through a hall opening into a comfortable lounge area. A coffee machine and a vending machine full of snacks sat against one wall so we got something to eat and drink and settled in for the long wait.

"Mr. and Mrs. Evans?" A tall young man in a dark suit approached, hand outstretched, "Doug Howard, hospital chaplain. Please don't get up," he said as Jeff moved to put down his magazine. "Enjoy your coffee. I wanted you to know, if you have the need to talk, I'm available. The chapel is a little way down the hall." We nodded then he smiled and walked out of the lounge.

"Come on, Kevin," I said. "Let's go and see the chapel." From what the chaplain had said, the room couldn't be far away. Kevin didn't put up any resistance. We found it a little way from the lounge, tucked in a corner and entered the tiny yet beautiful chapel. It seemed so peaceful and still that it invited those who yearned for spiritual guidance and consolation to enter.

While Kevin returned to sit with his father I sat alone inside the little church. I thought about this one surgical floor. I imagined the life and death decisions made here each day. As I prayed for my son's life to be spared, I recognized the immense value of this small chapel in its midst.

"Jan…Jan, wake up."

I don't know when I had fallen asleep. I'd left the chapel and gone back to the lounge to wait. Together we'd watched the hands of the clock move around the dial, ticking off the seconds. I raised my head to see Kevin in deep discussion with Doctor Newcomb. The hands of the clock appeared frozen at eleven-thirty.

"Is his operation over?" I asked.

The surgeon left Kevin and walked over to Jeff and me, giving us a weary grin. "The surgery went well but his vertebrae..." He shook his head. "It's a delicate procedure, like putting together bits and pieces of an intricate puzzle. We fixed two metal rods with screws on either side of the spine and..."

"Will he wake up...' I broke in.

"There's no change, Mrs. Evans. He's still in a coma. I've asked the neurologist to assess him as his recovery progresses. I can tell you he remains paralyzed from his waist down.

"When can we see him?" Kevin asked.

The doctor turned to face Kevin, "He'll be in the Recovery Room for some time. You folks might as well go home and try to get some sleep. All being well, Ron will be transferred from Recovery to the Surgical I.C.U. I would think not before mid-morning."

He's in a coma, paralyzed from the waist down. We made our way to the car without speaking and Kevin drove us home. I don't believe either Jeff or I could have managed it. Silent journey though it was, our silence said everything there was to say. Ron had survived and we had survived the darkest hours our family had ever known.

None of us could have imagined the hellish journey still ahead.

FIVE

Ron's surgery concluded, the days of waiting, not knowing the outcome, became our next challenge. Neither Jeff nor I dealt with this part well. Jeff's Home Care nurse visited every other day and George popped in from next door whenever he could. Kevin had flown back home leaving Jeff, his body weakened from the persistent infection, chafing at the extreme change in his routine.

I felt trapped. Torn between two opposing goals, I accomplished neither very well. While one pulled me in Ron's direction, the other pushed me toward Jeff and his need for support. My carefully constructed sense of order came crashing down one morning as I prepared for my usual tedious trip to the hospital.

"Where the hell did you hide my cereal bowl?" Jeff shouted from the kitchen.

"It's in the dishwasher. I didn't feel like taking the dishes out last night. Use another one," I mumbled, my mouth foaming with toothpaste and frustration.

"I can't find a damned thing in this kitchen anymore," he harangued, rattling dishes and cutlery.

My head started to throb again. Irritated by Jeff's petulant behaviour, I gargled, spit and turned off the faucet. Wrapped in my tatty bathrobe I marched down the hall. Fuming, I burst into the kitchen, retrieved Jeff's bowl from the dishwasher and flung it on the table. "There!" I said sharply. "I'm trying to get dressed. You could have waited..."

"Everything's going to hell in a hand basket," he complained as he shook cereal from its package into the bowl, indifferent to the mess he created. "Another phone call came from the hospital. You have a nine o'clock appointment."

"Nine?" I groaned. "Nine? I thought they said ten."

"What difference does it make?" Jeff bellowed. "Nine. Ten, who cares? What's so bloody urgent? He's in a coma, for God's sake. Why do you have to be there so early?"

With my hair a stringy mess, no makeup on and holding back tears, I screamed back at him. "Stop it, Jeff! Stop it! I can't stand your constant whining!" I felt the lump in my stomach rise up in my throat. I raced to the bathroom, shoved my head into the toilet bowl and threw up.

Jeff followed me into the bathroom. He

knelt on the floor behind me and held my head as I retched, spewing out all the anger, the ugliness, the absolute despair I had stuffed down and bottled up day after day.

He wiped my face and held me as we sat on the cold tiles. We rocked back and forth sobbing until there were no tears left. Without speaking, we stood up, wiped our faces and stumbled back into the family room to sit beside one another on the sofa.

"What's happening to us, Jan?"

My head drooped forward and my hair fell in front of my eyes. Jeff tenderly brushed it back. He put his hand under my chin and lifted up my head. I looked deep into the hazel eyes of the man I loved.

"Oh, my poor Jan. I'm so sorry. I didn't mean the things I said. I hate to think I blew my stack over a stupid cereal bowl, for Pete's sake. This morning, when I got up…oh, I don't know. I felt scared, afraid if you left the house, you might never come home again. Oh, honey, I've never been so afraid."

We're both afraid. We look at our beautiful son and we're afraid for his life, his future. We're fearful of the unknown, of a new and different tomorrow.

"I would never leave you, Jeff. I'm mixed up, too. You'll think I'm crazy when I tell you.

Everyone will think I'm crazy, but I need to know…"

"What? What is it?"

"I suppose I'm looking for answers, about his accident. What happened? Did he…how…oh, I feel so uncertain. I have thought about it though. I thought maybe…maybe we could hire a detective."

"Hire a detective, Jan? For goodness sake, why would we hire a detective?"

"Our own detective could investigate the accident. No one knows what happened for certain. The police didn't tell us much. They said alcohol and speed contributed to the crash. Maybe we won't learn anything different, but I'd like to try."

Jeff paused and then tapped his thin moustache, "A detective? Hmm…" His eyes widened. A deep chuckle began in his belly and grew until it burst out of him in a booming roar of laughter.

"You are so right, Jan. You are out of your mind. You're strap-you-into-a-strait-jacket crazy. Everyone will think you're loony-tunes but I love you to pieces. If hiring a detective to investigate the accident will ease your mind, then, by golly, that's what we're going to do!"

It was true. Jeff did love me, and he believed in me enough to back me up on this one.

"Okay. Now this is something I can do. You look after Ron and the hospital stuff, and I'll get on the computer and check out some agencies. You just leave everything to me."

"You're not joking? It would mean so much to me."

Hooking his thumbs into his belt, Jeff launched into a goofy movie cowboy routine, "Well shucks, little lady. Ah'd do anythin' fer a purty little gal like you."

Jeff's hilarious impersonations always made me laugh. When we looked at one another, we broke into laughter at the absurdity of it all. For those few minutes, everything felt right and normal again.

Outside, the morning air invigorated me. I hopped into the car, turned on the radio and hummed to the music coming from the FM station. As I drove along the smooth highway I relaxed into the soft leather upholstery of our new car. The white-capped mountains above Drydon offered a glorious backdrop to the city. I smiled as I thought of Jeff, busy at home digging into the mysteries of the detective business.

It seemed to me that the elevator to the Surgical I.C.U. had to be the slowest in the hospital. When the doors opened I looked out at a forbidding grey wall broken only by a single, thick pane of glass. Behind the glass sat a nurse whose bearing telegraphed her no-nonsense approach to unit security. The difference in the operation of this unit and the one Ron had been in before his surgery was dramatic. A red and white sign on the wall read, "SURGICAL I.C.U., AUTHORIZED STAFF AND THOSE ON VISITORS' LIST ONLY; VISITORS MUST PRODUCE I.D.; ONE VISITOR AT A TIME, PLEASE." Obediently, I opened my wallet, showed my I.D. and signed in before being buzzed into the ward.

Ron lay in his bed at the end of the long room. Tara, a sweet, young blond nurse, greeted me with a smile. She turned and introduced me to her male colleague.

"Good morning. Mrs. Evans, this is John, Ron's primary nurse. We're fitting your son with his body brace today."

John, a short muscular fellow with freckles and a shock of red hair, frowned down at the custom-fitted brace that held Ron's torso in its embrace. His speech confirmed my suspicion that he came from Scottish origin.

"I canna get the buckle tight enough, lassie. Could ye no' pull the strap further your way?" He glanced up at me and grinned. "G'mornin'. Nice to meet ye."

"Hello, John. How's my boy doing today?"

"We may see him off the ventilator soon, all goin' well." He checked the brace once more. Satisfied with their work, he nodded to Tara. She picked up their instruments and both left the bedside.

John's words of encouragement lifted my spirits. I looked around. Most of the patients in the room had suffered spinal injuries. Some, like Ron, also had brain injuries. I bent down to kiss my son but detected no response. I sighed and retrieved his washcloth and basin from the bedside cabinet, wiping around the brace as I gave him his morning sponge bath. When I finished I sat down, took one of his favourite stories from my bag and began to read aloud.

Tara walked over to the bed to note on her clipboard the information flashing and clicking from the machines around the bed. "Mrs. Evans, do you have a small radio at home?"

"Why, yes, I do Tara. Why do you…?"

"I noticed you talk to him all the time. I'm not sure if he hears you but maybe he does on some level. I thought if he enjoys music he could have a radio…"

"Of course, he'd love it. He knows all the bands. I'll bring one in tomorrow."

"Just a small one you understand. I think

some people respond to music and rhythm more than others. I'll be sure to turn it on softly. It will be put on his bedside table."

I hadn't thought about music. You never can tell.

Eight patients, four on each side of the bright room, occupied the beds, fitted out with an amazing array of life-saving paraphernalia. Some of the patients talked to the nurses, to one another or, feeling lonely, even to visitors.

"Hey, Mrs. Evans," called a rough but youthful voice from across the room.

I walked halfway toward the curtained cubicle. "How's everything with you this morning, Darren?" I called through the hospital drapery.

"It's the shits, Mrs. Evans," he returned with a mischievous laugh. "It's the shits."

"Don't ye pay any heed to that one," whispered John in confidence as he left the cubicle with an armful of dirty linen, "His talk's a wee bit crude this morning. That's his way of dealing with the situation but he'll learn."

Paralyzed. Of course they're all paralyzed. No one had talked to me in detail about the management of the bowel and bladder functions of a paralyzed person; nor had they discussed with me how Ron's spinal cord injury would affect that part of his daily life. I had supposed the subject would be dealt with later when our educational classes began.

I haven't really known a physically handicapped person, I realized. I remembered times when I had passed someone in a wheelchair, never giving a thought about where they found the strength, the courage to face their daily challenges.

I went back to Ron's bed. Why does his filthy hair bother me so much? I had washed his body as well as I could that morning but when I looked at his hair, still stiff from dried blood and caked with mud from the ditch where he'd been found, the pain in my gut returned. I wanted him back the way he used to be. I wanted him home in a familiar place where I could nag at him to get a haircut and keep his hair clean. My anger rose to the surface. I knew I wouldn't be satisfied until I could give him a shampoo.

"John, can you help me?"

Dressed as usual in his green scrubs, John bounded across the room. "What is it, Mrs. Evans? Is he all right?"

By the time John reached me, the tears streamed down my cheeks and I hiccupped, "His hair, John. I need to wash his hair."

"Now then, lass. I'll see what I can do. It'll no' be easy. But we'll manage, you wait and see. Sit yourself down. I'll be right back."

I had no idea what John had in mind but sank into a chair to wait. When John returned he carried two buckets, one filled with warm water and the other, empty.

"Now then, I'll shift him to the head of the bed and support his neck while you wash his head."

I contemplated the task ahead of us. I couldn't imagine how John's unique approach to the project would work. No wonder they hadn't washed his hair.

Somehow we managed. John held Ron's head and neck while I poured the water through his hair and into the empty bucket. I gagged when I saw the end result, one bucket of foul stinking muck. Although this shampoo couldn't compare with others I had given, still I felt much better.

"There ye are, lass," John murmured in his kind manner. He cleaned up the considerable mess and went back to his other duties.

To pretend Ron's hair had come out squeaky clean would have been ridiculous. But for the rest of the afternoon I hummed a favourite tune as I busied myself combing out the tangled mess. I considered for a moment cutting it all off but remembering the pride he took in his shoulder-length hair I thought better of it. Maybe later.

SIX

Jeff leaned back in his chair, put his feet up on the footstool and took a generous gulp of his evening cocoa. He hadn't said much during dinner but it didn't bother me. I'd been looking forward to a quiet evening anyway. Curled up on the sofa with my own double whipped cream version I sipped on my cocoa. I kicked off my fluffy slippers and wiggled my toes. After a long day with Ron I felt the need for comfort.

"Jeff?" A familiar voice hollered from outside the back door. Jeff looked over at me but I didn't make a move to get up so he swung his feet down from the stool and shuffled over to open the door for George.

The caked mud from his big boots scraped off on the doormat, George traipsed into the room and sat down backwards on a kitchen chair. "Can't stay, Jan," he said, his chin resting on the chair back. "Thought I'd come over and see if Jeff told you the news."

"What news? Jeff, what is it you haven't told me?"

My poker-faced husband looked up at the ceiling, rubbed his chin and chuckled, "Now, let me see. I know there was something…"

"Jeffrey Evans! What have you and George been up to now?"

George, who never could keep a straight face, roared with laughter. "It's the detective Jan," he said, as he wiped happy tears from his eyes. "Jeff and I have been working on it for over two weeks now and today…"

"Today, the detective…? What's happened?"

Jeff smiled and reached under his chair to pull out a heavy black binder. "It's all here Jan, photos and everything. We found this guy, well, George found him."

"No trouble at all," said George. "It all turned out fine, as it happened. I called this cop I used to know…"

Jeff interrupted, "…and he found this guy who used to be with the police force in Valleyview. Turned out he's had his own detective agency in Drydon for the past five years."

George slapped his thigh and got up to leave. "Got to go. Meeting's in half an hour." He turned and sauntered out the door, whistling an old tune.

I could have kissed them both for going to so much trouble but when Jeff placed the huge binder on my lap, I paused. The metal clasp of the book dug into my thighs. I felt uneasy.

The documents looked well-organized. I took note of the indexed subject files separated by coloured plastic dividers, and yet, I kept the clasp fastened as I imagined the serious burden awaiting anyone who opened it and read its pages.

I had begged Jeff to find someone who could discover what actually happened on that fateful night, someone who could find the answers to my nagging questions. It occurred to me as I held the unopened report that perhaps there are some questions best left unanswered. The knowledge the report contained might cause more grief than comfort but still, I ached to know. I took in a deep breath, opened the book and began to read. My desperate wish was that at the end of it all I might find some answers, even some hope.

The next morning I slept in. When I wandered out to the kitchen I found that Jeff had the coffee made and a bowl of cereal waiting for me on the kitchen table.

"Ah, just what I needed. Thanks honey. I don't know when I've slept so well."

"Yeah. I woke up about one o'clock. The light in the family room was still on so I figured you might still be reading. I didn't think you'd be in a hurry to get on the road."

"No, I'm not. It won't take me long to get ready, though. I'll be at the hospital in time for lunch."

Jeff looked at me from under his wrinkled brow. "What did you think of the report?"

"To be honest, Jeff, when I looked at the size of the binder, I felt overwhelmed."

"Me too, Jan. I thought we might read it a section at a time. We can talk about it as we go along."

"Mm...we could but when I noticed Mr. Jacobs' summary...you know me, I'm a lazy reader. I always turn to the last chapter first. So that's what I did last night."

"And...?"

"I read the summary. I looked over the diagrams and photographs. Oh, Jeff, I'm so grateful you and George found Mr. Jacobs."

"I should have stayed up with you last night. It must have been rough, going through those pictures by yourself." I heard the concern in my husband's voice and my mind returned to the night before when I had discovered some of the details of Ron's accident. Looking at the photos had been difficult. One view led me into the deserted, swampy field; the water-filled ditch where my son had been found, his head buried in the mud. The report indicated he had been unresponsive when discovered by the paramedics. They had resuscitated Ron at the site, manually bagged him, and kept him alive until they reached the hospital and connected him to a ventilator. Those caring, skilled people saved his life.

Some photos, released to our detective from police files showed skid marks indicating Ron had made an effort to correct his slide but failed. He had been driving too fast for the road conditions. Another showed different angles of the damaged vehicle. Gouges in the earth indicated the car had been airborne before it tumbled end-over-end, from the icy highway into the field. In one picture of the car's interior, I noticed an open vodka bottle sticking out from under the passenger seat. Empty beer bottles littered the floor of the car. According to one policeman, the vehicle reeked of alcohol. Ron's car keys still dangled from the ignition.

Ron's passenger had escaped injury. In one short paragraph, the police reported they had found him following the accident, stumbling about the field in such a drunken stupor it had been impossible for them to conduct an interview with him.

No one seemed to know anything about this fellow or where he and Ron may have gone after they left the McDonald's house. As

Jason told me, "He just turned up…a tall, skinny guy, older than us…"

I knew Jason's father would never have allowed Ron to drive away from their house drunk. I can only surmise that Ron, being a minor, had given his mystery passenger money to buy more alcohol which they both consumed prior to the accident. The police never did find Ron's wallet.

I arrived at the one question that had bothered me all along. How had his passenger escaped unhurt when Ron suffered such devastating injuries as the result of the same accident?The paramedics' report, along with police information discovered by our detective, Mr. Jacobs, held the answer. Upon examining Ron's body for injuries, no seatbelt marks appeared on his chest. Although the vehicle's airbags inflated, they had not saved Ron. When the front of the car, airborne and upended, first struck the ground, the doors had whipped open and Ron, his seatbelt unfastened, had been flung from the driver's seat into the air to land head down in the drainage ditch. His passenger, securely fastened in by his seat belt, had been saved from injury by the airbags.

It seemed ironic. The adult who purchased alcohol for Ron and his friends that night walked away unscathed while my son suffered the horrific consequences. That fact had always been difficult for me to accept. I decided that holding on to feelings of resentment, of ill will, toward someone whose identity I will never know will neither alter anything nor benefit anyone, especially me.

"It's all right, Jeff. At first I found the photos of his car upsetting. But the detective presented it all in such a professional, almost clinical fashion, it became easier to take after a while. I'm fine now, dear."

Jeff always made the best coffee. As I sat there breathing in its rich aroma, I realized for the first time since the accident, I'd found answers to some of the questions that had nagged at me for so long. I relaxed into the sofa with my coffee, smiled over at Jeff while a certain, delicious sense of family descended upon me.

When I walked into the I.C.U. that morning I sensed something different but I looked around and everything looked the same – the same patients occupied the same beds. The same nurses, busy as a hive of worker bees, flitted from bed to bed taking care of their charges and yet I felt a difference in the air.

Ron's bed sat at the end of the row lining the wall. When I reached him, I noticed he'd been propped against a pillow and was no longer on the ventilator.

"Come here, John," I called. "The head of Ron's bed is up. Did the doctor see him this morning?"

"Aye, came in about seven. Decided we could take him off the ventilator and prop him up. Don't fret. We're keeping an eye on him."

With Ron free of the breathing tube I sat listening as he breathed on his own for the first time since his accident. I should have rejoiced but a sense of unease kept niggling at me and I didn't know why.

I bent down to take a book from my bag. As I began to remove the bookmark I sensed Ron had moved. When first I glanced over at him I didn't notice a thing but as I lifted my head again, I heard it. A sound came from his lips, not words, but a peculiar mumble.

"John!" I cried. "I think he's trying to talk."

John strolled over to the bed and watched Ron's breathing for a bit. "It's his throat, Mrs. Evans. The breathing tube's left it a little raspy. But that'll ease…" Before John could finish his sentence Ron moved again. He threw his head back and moved it from side to side in perfect time to the music coming from his radio.

"Well, I'll be damned! Mrs. Evans, his eyes are open."

I pushed John aside to get a closer look at

Ron and his eyes were indeed, wide open. One of his eyes turned in toward his nose while the other stared straight ahead, as though unseeing. I stroked his arm and called his name but he neither saw me nor recognized my voice.

From somewhere deep inside his poor bruised brain erupted his youthful response to a popular song coming from his bedside radio. "Rock rocks!" he shrieked, lifting his arm in a kind of adolescent salute. He tossed his head back again, turned it from side to side and howled like a scalded wolf.

I didn't care about the noise. I shouted; I wept for joy. Tara raced over to see what happened. Amidst smiles and tears word of the awakening spread throughout the ward like a contagion. Ron had finally come to and everyone joined in the celebration. He didn't recognize anyone or anything. Though his eyes had opened I knew he couldn't see but he had spoken. I couldn't wait to phone home.

"Hello, Jeff. Wait until I get my breath! I had to use the phone at the desk. My cell phone doesn't work in here."

"Slow down Jan and don't yell. I can't understand you. What did you say about your cell phone?"

"No. Not my cell phone. It's Ron Jeff, he woke up. He even said a couple of words, but…"

Jeff didn't let me finish. "You stay right where you are. I'll catch a cab. George isn't home. Wow! I think I'm going to kiss you right through the damned phone."

"Jeff, he doesn't recognize anyone. He won't know who you are."

"Who the hell cares? The kid's come to. They've got therapists. It'll take time, that's all."

"Of course. It'll take time. Yes, you're right, Jeff. See you soon."

My husband almost bounded into the ward this time. "Ronny," he said, leaning over to hug his son. Ron didn't move.

"He's fallen asleep."

"That's okay," Jeff replied as he kissed Ron's limp hand. "He really talked? You heard him?"

"Oh yes. Everyone heard him but he hasn't moved in the past while."

John came over to put Ron's bed back down. "Mustn't overdo on his first day," he reminded us as he straightened the bed sheets.

"It's been a great day, eh, John?"

"Aye, Mr. Evans. Glad you could make it. The boy's given us a pleasant surprise today." Jeff nodded, grinned with pride and turned his attention back to Ron.

"His colour's better. I'd hoped he'd still be awake when I got here."

John glanced over at me. "He's had his medication, Mr. Evans," he said. "I expect he'll sleep the night away now. Your son's had a long day. It's been a bit of a strain for him sitting up for the first time and…"

"I know. Jan told me. He opened his eyes and talked today. I couldn't believe my ears when she called."

"It's been a grand day for us all. He's not alert yet. It'll be a wee while…"

I interrupted them. "Jeff, he's sleeping now. In the morning when I get here, if he's awake I'll call you in right away. We should probably go now. It is getting late."

"Yeah, poor guy, he's all tuckered out. Okay, let's get some dinner in the cafeteria and go home."

The next day brought another surprise. Doctor Newcomb had been in and ordered Ron's feeding tube removed.

"Lunchtime," called the kitchen aide as she placed Ron's meal of beef broth and some kind of juice on his tray. "Are you feeding him his lunch today, Mrs. Evans?" she asked. I nodded and she left to deliver another patient's meal. A new sign above Ron's bed read, FEED. FLUIDS ONLY. He could not feed himself.

I wrapped a towel around Ron's neck to catch the drips and dribbles. As a mewling kitten would do, he moved his head back and forth searching blindly for his food. He stuck his tongue out to touch the spoon I held in my hand, slurped at the contents, pursed his lips together and swallowed. His tongue rolled around in his mouth for a while as if he enjoyed the taste. With his tongue curled up beneath his nose, he inhaled the smell of the food.

I realized we had both been here before. As an infant, he had searched for his bottle and fed in the same way. I believed Ron had found a way to learn.

Christmas came and Christmas went. It had been three weeks since Ron's surgery; a whole month since the accident. I couldn't recall much of my annual trip to the mall in search of gifts but I must have shopped and wrapped the presents because there they sat, under the tree. Jeff and Kevin decorated the tree and I prepared our traditional Christmas Eve dinner. Although brightened by Kevin's presence, the holiday felt like one big blur.

"Mom," Kevin said, a few days after Christmas, "are you and Dad planning to take some time out for yourselves any time soon?"

"Kevin!" I protested, as I bustled about

clearing the dinner table. "What a question. We can't leave Ron. We haven't time for a vacation right now; not until he's well again."

"Yeah?" His tone had undergone a change. "How long will it take until he's well again? Six months, a year maybe? I've talked it over with Dad and he's worried about you, Mom."

"Don't be silly Kevin. Everything's fine. You saw Ron the other day. Didn't you think he'd improved?" I asked as I plumped up the sofa cushions, avoiding his piercing gaze.

Why must he follow me with his eyes? I fumed to myself. He's making me nervous.

"Yeah, I saw him Mom. At least I saw someone who looks like my brother but it isn't him. Yeah, you're right. Someone will be coming home sooner or later but it won't be Ron. It will be a far different person who comes through that door." His words cut like a knife and my whole body began to shake.

Jeff walked in from the garage in time to catch the last part of Kevin's remarks. He walked over and put his arm around my shoulder and squeezed. "She knows, Kevin. Deep down, she knows. You don't have to remind her. She's his mother, for God's sake. Give her a break."

Jeff's arm tightened around me as he noticed my stricken expression. "Moms don't give up on their kids, Kevin. On the other hand, guys, yeah, guys like you and me – I don't think we'd have the backbone to carry the load your mother has for all these weeks."

Kevin swiped his hand across his runny nose as tears ran down his cheeks. "I'm sorry Mom. I'd like to see you and Dad get away from all this for a while, that's all."

Still shaking, I took Kevin's hand and we sat side-by-side on the sofa as I pulled my knees up to my chin and wept. I realized I had allowed Ron's care to take over my whole life. It had occupied my time and all my thoughts to the exclusion of everyone and everything else. It wasn't fair and it had to stop. Oh, not the caring for Ron. That had to continue but perhaps at a more measured pace. I decided to take Kevin's advice to heart and give us all a break.

"I'd love to take a holiday with Dad, Kevin but I don't think we would enjoy it if we didn't have someone here who Ron knows; someone who would visit him while we're away." I thought for a moment then sighed. "A short cruise does sound tempting though, doesn't it, Jeff?"

Kevin jumped up. "Okay. Okay, it's a deal. I have some vacation time saved up. Will you two promise to go on a cruise if I can stay here and look after Ron?"

Kevin flew back home the next day. That evening we received a phone call from him, "Hi Mom. I'm calling to let you know I can take a week off next month. So, if you can book a cruise I'll come home and look after Ron."

And so we did.

SEVEN

"Hurry up, Jan. I see a couple of deck chairs over there."

Our heads bowed down against the cold wind, Jeff and I pushed through the heavy doors that opened onto the deck. We wanted to find a good spot to enjoy the celebration as our ship cruised out of the harbour. Jeff had pointed out a nice viewing place and we raced to claim our chairs.

"Wait here. I'm going over to the bar and get some coffee."

"Double-double whipped cream for me, Jeff."

"Would you like a blanket ma'am?" offered the smiling steward.

"We'll need two, please. My husband will be coming back."

I took one blanket and placed it on the back of Jeff's deck chair and wrapped myself in the other. With a deep sigh, I snuggled down, kept my eyes on the railing in front me and waited for Jeff to return. A lively band on deck began to play a familiar tune and my feet twitched and tapped in time to the music. I looked away from the railing for a moment to see Jeff hurrying back with our drinks.

"Here you are, honey," he said, smiling as he handed me my coffee and sank into his chair. "Double whipped cream, as usual."

The setting sun became a fiery ball on the horizon, adding to the festive mood. With a mighty blast from its horn the huge ship began to move.

Other passengers lined the rails, threw streamers and waved to people on the dock below. Small boats in the harbour joined in as they blew their whistles, saluting the big ship as it sailed past. Settled beneath the blankets with our hands cupped around steaming coffee cups, we leaned back and watched in contentment as the skyline of the city disappeared from view.

Overnight our ship made its way south into warmer waters and we exchanged our winter clothing for summer wear. As we packed away our heavy jackets the emotional weight we had both been carrying dropped away. We cruised and spoiled ourselves for a few days then docked and took a little yellow bus through low-lying hills to our luxurious hotel.

"This is the life, eh, Jan?"

"What shall we do first? I'd like to visit the shops for some of the up-to-date fashions they have here."

"I thought we agreed to get away from it all, Jan. Seems that didn't include getting away from your trips to the shopping malls."

"I promise I won't overdo the shopping. We should look for some souvenirs to take home, though," I countered.

Our vacation flew by. Because of his heart condition, Jeff couldn't walk far so we rented scooters, saw the sights, shopped, and lost more money than we intended playing the slot machines.

"Jan!" Jeff called from the bathroom on the last evening of our vacation. "Our flight's at nine tomorrow. I hope you've packed."

I had stuffed brochures, tickets and other mementos of our trip into my carry-on bag. "I'm way ahead of you," I answered. "I have already put our bags in the hall for pickup. Let's get a good night's sleep." I yawned, turned down the bedcovers and crawled into bed.

Jeff jumped in the other side of the bed and leaned over to kiss me, "G'night hon. We had a great time, didn't we?"

"The best, Jeff," I said with a deep, satisfied sigh. "The very best."

Our first visit with Ron after we arrived home amazed us. For one thing, he could see.

Whether he understood what he saw, I didn't know. He had progressed to eating solid food. I noticed he moved about more and I could swear the peculiar sounds he made had some meaning. Although I could have done without the strange howling noise that came out of nowhere for no apparent reason, I was thrilled by his progress.

A large metal rack stacked with hospital linen stood against the wall near his cubicle. Propped up in bed, Ron faced the wall and muttered to himself. His head and arms jerked up and down. He appeared to be frustrated about the metal linen rack for some reason.

"I can't figure it out, John," I said to his attending nurse. "I think he's trying to do some work and he's confused. See the way he's moving his head and arms? Look how he's curling his fingers. It's as though he's trying to write."

"I wouldn't think so. We'll see. Wait here and I'll be right back."

John strode over to the nursing station, gathered some items and returned with a notepad and pencil. When he placed the pencil between Ron's fingers, he held onto it with a firm, precise grip.

"Well, I'll be...you could be right. I'll leave the notepad here. See what the lad can do wi' that."

I placed the notepad in Ron's other hand. With the same cross-eyed stare as before, he shot me a strange, lopsided grin. His muttering lessened and his movements became more deliberate. While his head continued to bob up and down, there seemed to be some purpose to his efforts. His movements had a certain rhythm to them. When he touched his pencil to the paper, he shouted in excitement. I couldn't see anything but scribbles on the paper and when his pencil slipped off the paper, he continued to make the same scribbles on the bed cover. I felt his actions had something to do with his work; something he'd been doing on the day before his accident.

When I got home later, I still couldn't get the notion out of my mind. "Jeff," I yelled as I came in the door. "Let's go down to the warehouse."

"What warehouse? I thought we were going out for dinner tonight."

"I meant let's go to the warehouse in the morning," I said, as I tossed my purse on the table.

"Okay, Jan. You've got me. Where are we going tomorrow?"

"To Ron's work, Conrad Plumbing Supplies," I replied, rolling my eyes. "We have the detective's report about the accident itself, but

I don't think we'll find the answer there. I'm sure it has something to do with his job."

"Answer to what? You're not making a whole lot of sense right now," he said as he helped me take off my coat. I relayed what had happened during my visit with Ron.

"You could be on to something. I wouldn't mind taking a day off from all this cooking and cleaning anyway," he said, pretending to wipe sweat from his forehead. "All right, we'll go down to Conrad's in the morning."

Early the next day Jeff and I drove to the warehouse where Ron had last worked. Sandra, the secretary, had taken our early call. A self-assured, long-legged young woman, she greeted us as we walked in to her second-floor office. "It's good to see you two," she said, shaking our hands. As she talked she twisted her tawny blond ponytail into a knot and pinned it on top of her head. "My hair gets in the way, working in this place," she explained. "How's Ronny doing?"

"Coming along, Sandra," Jeff answered. "We came down to see if we could find out exactly what he was doing before he left work the day of his accident."

"Oh, that's easy. He was taking inventory."

"Taking inventory? Do you think we could go down to the warehouse and look around?" I asked.

"No problem. We'll have to stay out of the way of the forklift though," she said as she led us down a steep flight of stairs to the main floor of the building.

When we stepped into the massive warehouse, I felt a cold draft coming from the open loading bay. We hadn't walked too far when I stopped and tugged at Jeff's arm, "There it is Jeff. That's what Ron's been looking at."

In front of us stood row upon and row of metal racks filled with the company's products. What I had witnessed in the I.C. U. had been Ron, his eyes fixed upon the metal linen rack facing him, trying to count the products he imagined were stacked there. He had been attempting to take inventory, the same job he'd been doing on his last day of work. He remembered the day of his accident.

I began to cry and Jeff put his arms around me, "You're right, Jan. Ron's in there somewhere. We just have to find a way to reach him."

I continued to sit beside Ron each day. I talked to him and did the same things we'd done for weeks but could see no further improvement.

"Tara. What more I can do? I feel like we've reached a dead end."

"You could begin with a scrapbook. If he had pictures to look at, pictures of people he knows, familiar things, he may begin to remember, to name them. I think it would be worth a try."

That evening I started Ron's scrapbook. It was more like a photo album with pictures of family, friends, his pets and ordinary household objects. I printed names underneath each one. Armed with our "Big Book", as I called it, I began my own homegrown style of speech therapy.

When first he began to speak his words emerged garbled and meaningless. But as we progressed, I felt they held meaning, though he continued to reverse or scramble them. The Big Book proved to be a success when Ron began to bang his hand down on a certain page, grunt, and then bang his hand down again. He refined his actions and started to point his finger to a person or object when it took his fancy. One day while I flipped through the pages of the book, he grabbed my hand and forced me to stop. He pointed to a picture of his kitten, Fluffy. He looked sad as he put his face down against the picture and said, "Ah..." as tears rolled down his cheeks.

I wept along with him and choked out the name, Fluffy. He looked at me, struggled, and repeated, "Foolf." He had recognized and named the subject of one of the photos.

Moving rapidly from that point, he pointed at and named in his own peculiar language most of the photos in his book. I thought he'd begun to recognize Jeff and me. One day when Jeff came to visit him he reached up, pulled his father's head down to meet his and said, "Ad, ur Ad."

That was good enough for Jeff. "He knows me," he wept. "He knows me, Jan."

One morning a few weeks later when I entered the ward, I was horrified to hear a string of curses along with the usual howls and shrieks, coming from my son's mouth. Tara went about her duties as usual acting as though she hadn't noticed.

I took John aside to discuss this turn of events. "Aye, lass, that's common behaviour for some with brain injuries. Listen to that one, will ye."

He drew my attention to the bed opposite Ron's. There, a teen-aged girl, another motor vehicle accident victim tried her best to match Ron's colourful speech with her own. The swearing contest between the two continued throughout the day. After a while I covered my ears in a vain effort to silence the profanity.

I noticed the anguished looks on the faces

of the couple visiting the young girl and walked across the room to introduce myself, "Hi there. My name's Janice Evans. The boy in the bed across from you is my son."

"Your son, oh, you poor dear," the woman cried. "I'm Ethel, Ethel Jamieson. This is my husband, Frank, and this…," she said, pointing to the girl in the bed, "…this is my daughter, Jennifer."

We all cringed as another spate of foul language gushed from Jennifer's rosy little mouth.

Frank lifted his head up from his hands and said, "This isn't like her. She's never uttered a bad word in her life. We're a Christian family. I don't know…"

"That's alright, Frank. It's all new to me as well."

"Your son…," said Frank.

"…a car accident."

"The same as happened to our Jennifer. Driving home from grad their car went over a cliff."

As the day wore on the deafening noise and objectionable language coming from the two young people showed no sign of stopping.

"I wonder if you would like to join me for an early supper," I said to the couple.

"That would be lovely, wouldn't it, Frank?" Ethel replied. Frank nodded in silence, too distraught to speak. The three of us left our rambunctious, potty-mouthed teen-agers in the capable hands of a new and fresher shift of nurses while we had dinner and compared notes in the cafeteria.

In spite of the obvious problem with Ron's constant cursing, I felt he'd made real progress. Though he reversed and garbled his words and sentences, when angry or upset his language became clearer, more understandable. I thought I'd ask Jeff what he thought.

"I'd like to get an appointment with one of the neurologists. The way he's progressing, someone should be able to give us a better idea of what we can expect in the future."

Jeff frowned, "I don't know, Jan. Maybe it's too soon to tell. He's like a young child in so many ways."

"But maybe they should be starting him on more advanced therapy. I'm a complete amateur when it comes to this stuff. I haven't any idea what I'm doing half the time."

"You're doing your best. Look how Ron's advanced. What could be better than to have his own mother teach him? It isn't as if you haven't done it before,"

"I'm not so sure. I'd like to find out if there's something more to be done. It wouldn't hurt to ask."

"Okay. But don't get your hopes up."

I asked Doctor Newcomb, who visited Ron regularly if he would contact the neurology department and arrange for a consultation. He agreed and, although Doctor Fieldman wouldn't be available, his assistant booked an appointment for me with another neurologist for the following week.

The day I had been waiting for arrived. The elevator rose in its usual slow fashion to the floor above the I.C.U. As the doors opened I noticed a receptionist peering out from behind her glass window.

"My name is Mrs. Evans. I have an appointment…"

"Yes, Mrs. Evans," she said before I had a chance to say more. "You are in Meeting Room Four. It's down the hall and to your left."

"Thank you," I said, and began the walk down the long corridor. Where one hallway met the other, I turned left as instructed. Room Four turned out to be about another block away. I walked through the open door into a cold, empty room. The furniture looked the same as other hospital meeting rooms, with a black metal desk and two chairs. The obligatory box of tissues and a full pen holder sat on the desk. I perched on one of the chairs, put my purse on my lap and waited.

A pale blond man dressed in a conservative grey suit entered with a thick file tucked in the crook of his arm. I knew my favourite neurologist, Doctor Fieldman, wouldn't be there to see me because he'd be away at a conference. I would miss his warm smile. Not only did this man in front of me not smile, he seemed aloof, even cold.

He didn't introduce himself but sat down across the desk from me, opened his file and looked down at his watch. Oh, oh, I thought, suddenly worried. He's impatient, as well.

When he stood up he clicked a switch to light up the panels fixed to the wall. He leaned back and using a pointer, indicated certain peculiar blotches on the x-rays. I supposed they were of Ron's head but he didn't explain. The young doctor spouted out such a stream of professional language, I couldn't even follow him. I clutched the handle of my purse as he rose to leave.

"Yes, doctor," I said, finally. "I wanted to know what you thought of my son's progress. He's been doing so well lately and…"

He gave me no opportunity to finish my thought but sat back down in complete silence. He swiped off his rimless glasses and proceeded to polish them while his eyes dropped down to the file in front of him. He replaced his glasses on his nose and looked across the desk at me.

"Mrs. Evans, Ronald has suffered severe brain damage in addition to the injury to his spine. There is little hope he can be managed at home. My suggestion at this point would be to put his name on the list for a long-term care placement following his discharge from hospital."

"You can't mean a permanent nursing home, for Ron? But…but," I stammered, thinking about my son's recent improvement.

"What I'm trying to say, Mrs. Evans is that it is possible your son will remain a vegetable for the rest of his life."

I felt a surge of anger. I wanted to leap across the desk, take this man by the throat and make him swallow his words. I wanted to curse him and the whole professional establishment but I stopped to remember the two young people lying in their beds in the I.C.U. whose curses could put my efforts to shame. I knew they'd be more than able to express my feelings if they were here in my place.

Had he said what I thought he said or was my imagination playing tricks on me? Confused, I glanced at the doctor. I turned and looked around me. Had I wandered into the wrong meeting room by mistake? Whatever the case, the phrase, "…a vegetable," rang in my ears. It made me more determined than ever to find a way to help Ron recover as much as possible from his injuries. If this guy's trying to practice some kind of reverse psychology on me, I think it's working, I thought as I gathered my purse handles and stood up.

"Well, thank you for your time, doctor," I said before I left the room. When I reached the hallway I looked back. He had vanished and I realized I might never know the name of this man in the grey suit who held out no hope for my son.

EIGHT

Ron acted so child-like I was reminded of his younger years. Images of him as a youngster ran through my mind like old home movies. In spite of what the neurologist had said I thought there had to be something someone could do to help Ron but, where to start?

"It's always best to begin at the beginning…," I'd heard and so we began, at the beginning.

"What's that ye've brought in with ye today?"

I held up a plastic crate. "It's a toy box, John. The scrapbook has been a great help, but I thought if Ron had something he could touch and feel as well as see, his language skills might improve more."

John chuckled. "Ye never cease to amaze me."

My husband called me a 'pack rat' but I knew there had to be a good reason I'd kept some of the boys' old playthings. Within a short time Ron began to hold and name his favourite toys. He held his beat up toy cars in his fist, made engine sounds, and drove them up and down the hills and valleys of his hospital bedspread. Whenever he felt tired he'd reach for his tattered old bear, tuck it under one ear and go to sleep.

One morning I walked into the I.C.U. as usual and walked over to his bed. It was empty.

"Tara! Where's Ron?"

"Oh dear, didn't they phone you? He's been moved to a regular ward, Room 212, Bed 3."

He's been promoted! "But…how…?" I stammered.

"He's well enough physically to be on the ward. Doctor Newcomb took him off the intensive care list."

"What about his meals? He's still not feeding himself, or..."

"He'll find plenty of help on the ward. The company of the other young men should do him some good."

Blinking back tears of joy, I hugged the grinning I.C.U. staff one by one, gathered up Ron's belongings and went to look for him. As soon as I heard the familiar howl, I knew his room couldn't be far away. Although his cursing had lowered a few decibels, for some reason, his awful screeching and howling continued. I wondered how long his new roommates would put up with the racket. As it turned out, the answer was, not for long.

"Shut up, Ron!" I heard a young male voice yell out from across the room.

"Ron! Hush, be quiet," I scolded him.

The noise stopped. "Ma!" he babbled, "Ma, car!"

I reached into the crate I had brought from the I.C.U, and took out one of his cars. When I placed it in his hand, he felt it, brought it close to his eyes and laughed. "Ha-Ha, ur car. Brrum, brrum." He pushed that little car up and down all around the bed then he threw back his head and howled some more.

"Mrs. Evans?" a deep velvety voice spoke over the din. I turned to see a tall, black male nurse smiling down at me. "My name's Earl. I'm Ron's primary care nurse."

"Ah, yes. I'm Ron's mother. I'm so sorry. I haven't any idea why he makes that awful noise. Is he settling in well otherwise?"

The man broke into a hearty laugh. "He's doing fine. But the rest of these guys didn't get much sleep last night."

"He started making those noises in the I.C.U. He didn't respond at all until one of the nurse suggested I bring in the radio..."

Earl rubbed his chin. "Mm...the radio. I've got an idea, Mrs. Evans. Mind if I try something?"

"I'm ready to try anything," I moaned as Ron turned his head from side-to-side and howled again. "The noise drives me crazy, too."

"Okay, let's try this." Earl reached over to the head of Ron's bed and turned off the radio.

"Now listen." He turned to face the other patients. "Anybody hear anything now?"

"Hey! What did you do, Earl?" asked the boy in the next bed.

I felt a heavenly silence descend upon the room. "He isn't howling anymore."

The nurse reached over and turned the radio back on. An ear-splitting, wolf-like howl sounded throughout the ward.

"Stop that damned noise!" shouted one of the boys.

Earl scratched his head and again turned off the music, "I knew there had to be a trigger. Something set him off to make those noises. It's funny. As soon as I heard him I had a hunch he'd been trying to sing."

"Sing?" the other boy snorted. "You call that singing?"

I felt foolish. Of all the members of our family, Ron was the only one who couldn't hold a tune. He'd always loved listening to music, especially rock, but whenever he tried to join in and sing everyone covered their ears.

Our nurse, Tara, had been on the right track when she suggested giving him the radio. He had responded but not as anyone could have imagined. We had assumed the peculiar sounds he made had something to do with his brain injury. Not so. My tone-deaf son had been trying to sing along with the music he heard on the radio. Other patients on the ward nicknamed him "The Karaoke Kid" but the staff got tough and limited his radio time.

Ron's speech continued to improve but his memory didn't. One day, when Doctor Newcomb made his rounds he stopped at the bedside. "Hi, Ron, remember me?" The doctor's question met with a smile and Ron's usual blank, cross-eyed stare. He didn't recognize the doctor he had seen almost every day since his admission to hospital. His short-term memory had been seriously impaired by the brain injury. Although he used more words every day, he interrupted his garbled speech with strange hiccup-like yelps.

Jeff came with me whenever he could. Together we attended instructional classes designed to help patients and their families deal with injuries like Ron's. Each patient had a manual, one for Brain Injury and the other for Spinal Cord Injury. We received one of each. Jeff and I studied them during quiet evenings.

Ron's eyes didn't focus well enough to read but we hoped that reading would come later.

Ron and his roommates all looked forward to their promotion to Drydon Rehabilitation Centre, situated a few blocks away from the main hospital. As I watched the others move toward their goal, I couldn't help but compare Ron's dismal progress to theirs.

Each patient's injuries differed from those of another. The level of spinal cord injury determined the degree of disability suffered. Diagnosed a paraplegic, Ron's spinal cord had been severed at waist level. He had full use of his upper torso and arms but not his legs. A couple of the other fellows in the room had sustained higher level injuries that affected the use of their arms as well as their legs. They were diagnosed as quadriplegic. One young man, Eric, had broken his neck in a car accident. His was the highest level of spinal cord injury one could sustain and still survive. His head and neck were fixed within a device called a 'halo'. He had little use of his arms or legs. He couldn't transfer on his own, so the hospital aides used a sling attached to his bed to transfer him from bed to wheelchair. He would need a personal attendant to care for him for the remainder of his life.

To a one, the young men I met in Room

212 displayed an unexpected spirit of grace and humour considering their appalling situations. I admired their courage, especially those who had no family support. With sadness, I recalled the statistics cited by one of the doctors: "The majority of spinal cord injuries occur among males between the ages of eighteen and twenty-four." Not one of these brave young men wanted to remain in the hospital. They worked hard so they could progress to the rehabilitation centre and from there into the community.

"Bye, Ron. Bye Mrs. Evans. See you when you get to the Centre," they would say, as one by one they transferred to their new home. As Ron's roommates left so his eagerness to follow them grew. The day finally came when Earl brought a wheelchair to the bedside. "All right, boy, time to get you moving out of here."

The tricky balancing act of transferring from bed to wheelchair began. When Ron first got the hang of wheeling the chair, he moved back and forth within the confines of the ward. But as he gained confidence and speed, in his cross-eyed, wobbly fashion, he headed for the door.

"Look out. Here he comes!" a staff member yelled one afternoon as he leapt out of the way of the weaving wheelchair coming toward him at full speed down the corridor.

"I'm so sorry. He's not used to steering yet," I apologized. As a result of his head injury Ron had little impulse control. He couldn't visualize himself or his chair in relation to the space he occupied or the speed the wheelchair traveled. No wonder the staff all keep so fit, I thought.

With my shins painfully sore from repeated run-ins with the chair, I limped along behind him to his remedial classes. These included speech and language therapy, occupational therapy as well as training in bladder and bowel routines. That was only the beginning. I don't know how much of it Ron took in but I knew we both had a great deal more to learn.

"Jeff, I don't know if Ron will ever manage this stuff by himself. My head is aching after a day like today. He's booked for one therapy session after another."

"It's time you took a break. Ron doesn't need you there every day. If you're not there, someone will look after him. The sooner he learns he can't depend on you for everything, the better."

"But he needs me… his meals, his classes. I have to be there to remind him when it's time to get ready, help him into his chair…"

"Jan! Ron is the one who needs to remember, not you. As long as you're there telling him what to do and when, he doesn't have to try. I've watched him. He gets in and out of that chair fine all by himself."

I felt my face getting red. "You have no idea what it's like for him, Jeff, or for me. Everything is so difficult."

My body started to heave with sobs. "My son's body is broken into pieces and I don't know how to fix it!"

Jeff tried to put his hand on my shoulder but I twisted away from him.

"That's it exactly Jan. You can't fix it. He's my son too, remember. I think you need to allow the hospital staff to do their jobs. What that boy needs is professional help. You and I don't have the training."

I turned my back on him. As I trembled with anger I plopped down on the sofa. I grabbed a nearby cushion and pushed it deep into my midsection as if my insides would all spill out if I didn't hold them in.

"What do you mean, you and I? How often are you there to help him?"

"Careful Jan, you're tired. You know you say things you don't mean when you're upset."

I reached for a tissue, blew my nose and wiped away hot tears of resentment. I disregarded my husband's advice and went to bed unhappy. The next morning I left the house without saying goodbye to him.

When Ron's transfer to Drydon Rehabilitation Centre came through I arrived at the centre bright and early, ready to meet him, to help him get settled when he arrived but Ron didn't seem too pleased to see me. He sat in his chair with his arms crossed and glared at me from across the foyer. He resents me being here, I realized with a shock. At that moment I thought about Jeff and how miserably I had treated him lately. I thought now how valid his assessment of Ron's situation had been. I suddenly recognized that, as our son gained back his sense of self, his male ego had been threatened by my smothering.

For some reason this situation reminded me of a day following Ron's third birthday. We had been walking along the sidewalk. I bent down to take him by the hand. His little face reddened with anger as he twisted his small hand out of mine and stated in a firm voice, "I'm free years ode. Let go! I can do it by myself!"

As I drove home from the rehabilitation centre I couldn't hold back the tears. I thought about the terrible things I had said to Jeff. My tires screeched as I swerved into our driveway. I slammed the car door and ran into the house.

"Jeff. Jeff, are you home?" I felt terrible that once again I had become so engrossed in Ron's care that I had neglected Jeff and the rest of my family. He wandered out from the bathroom drying his hands.

"What's up? I heard the car. You shouldn't take that turn so fast."

I fell into his arms and sobbed. "Oh honey. I'm sorry I didn't listen to you. I don't know what is the matter with me."

Jeff's arms held me tight. "It's okay, sweetheart. It's okay. I understand. I couldn't have stopped you anyway, not until you felt ready. You're his mother, for God's sake. Sometimes you act like a mother bear protecting her cub."

"But what you said about Ron and me was true. He must learn to do more for himself. He doesn't want me there all the time. I've decided to cut my visits down to a couple of days a week."

"Great," said Jeff, rubbing his whiskers against my soggy cheek. "It'll be good to have you home more often. You don't know how much I've missed you." He stepped back, turned me around and grinned. "Wadda ya say we step out for dinner and a movie, kid?"

I sighed with relief. "Only if you shave off that beard."

I didn't wake up until almost ten o'clock the

next morning. I got up, stretched and flopped back down on the bed. Still full of remorse, I thought how I had allowed myself to backslide, to live in my own selfish "mother zone". I hadn't stopped to consider how Ron's accident and my reaction to it had impacted upon our marriage and upon our entire family. Ron's life had not been the only one broken into pieces by that car accident.

NINE

"I'll meet you here at lunchtime," I said.

Ron turned and waved. I watched as he wheeled down the hall of the rehabilitation centre to attend another therapy session. I knew he would be gone for at least an hour so I strolled over to a snug corner of the foyer to wait. I sank down into one of the yellow leather sofas, bent down and pulled a book from my shoulder bag. The sun twinkled among the branches of the ancient maples guarding the entrance and streamed through the ceiling-high windows. Caught by a sudden spring breeze, the trees swayed creating leafy shadow patterns on the polished marble floor. The centre bustled with activity. A constant parade of patients, staff and visitors passed through it. I tried to imagine their personal stories and where they were going in such a hurry. With so many interesting things to draw my attention, my book slipped unread into my lap. I leaned back and relaxed as I contemplated the busy scene passing before me.

Fewer visits from me during the week had a positive effect upon Ron. As time passed, I felt more comfortable with my decision. His sense of independence improved without me hovering about, supervising his every move.

"Follow me," he called out one day as he sped through the maze of hallways. He whipped around corners to show me the various therapy rooms and stopped to talk to staff members. His face lit up each time a lovely female staffer crossed our path. He certainly hasn't changed much in that regard, I thought ruefully.

Ron had been placed on the Brain Injury floor of the Drydon Centre with older brain injured patients. Most had suffered strokes. Ron and I felt disappointed he hadn't been sent to the same ward as the young men he'd met during his hospital stay. "Rick, Ken, where?" he'd ask. "Ode man," he sulked, pointing to his elderly roommate whose conversation skills lagged behind his own.

Two of his friends from Room 212, Rick and Ken, had been sent to the ward for those with spinal cord injuries. Some had been injured in vehicle accidents, others in work-related mishaps. Ron faced a dilemma. He suffered from both head and spinal injuries. He didn't fit in well with clients on either ward.

I took a deep breath. I tried to hold my head high as I approached the pretty receptionist in the foyer. "I'm Ron Evans' mother. I'd like to make an appointment with one of the team looking after my son."

"Oh, I know Ron well." Her brown eyes twinkled, "My name's Ellen. Ron comes to visit me every day."

Oh, oh…he's been flirting with this girl as well.

I smiled and began again, "I'm not sure who it is I should see. I'm concerned about his ward placement. There aren't any people there his age."

"I can look after that for you." Ellen consulted her computer. "Yes, Charlotte Gordon has an opening this afternoon. Could you be here for a two o'clock appointment?"

"Thanks, Ellen. I'll be back at two," I replied, delighted to be seen so soon.

We had plenty of time for lunch. When Ron and I got in the cafeteria lineup, I had to steel myself not to help him with his food. I noticed most of the other clients tried to manage for themselves, although it did take them more time and effort than others. A couple of the young men, quadriplegics, needed help with feeding. One had been fitted with a leather wristband with a device attached to hold his cutlery. With the help of an attendant he tried over and over to get the food onto his fork and up to his mouth. Most of it landed back on his plate or on the floor. When he did succeed in getting a mouthful, his face lit up with pride and he dug into his food with renewed purpose. Off in one corner all by themselves sat an elderly couple. From what I could see the husband had suffered a stroke. He couldn't feed himself. I noticed the woman's withered hand tremble as she held a spoonful of soup up to her husband's mouth. After he swallowed as much as he could, she wiped the dribbles from his mouth and chin. In what seemed a fit of frustration, he yelled at her and knocked the spoon out of her hand. How will she manage when he goes home? I wondered, feeling for her distress.

Rick and Ken spotted Ron and motioned for us to join them. "When are you moving up to our floor, Ron?"

"G'morrow," Ron shouted, adding a couple of sharp yelps. Everyone at the table jumped at his shrill cries but he seemed unaware.

"Yay," laughed Ken. "Be sure to leave your radio at home. If you start singing again we'll tape your mouth shut." I hoped he'd be rooming with one of these great guys but we'd have to wait and see.

After lunch, I met Charlotte Gordon at the reception desk and she led me to her office on the main floor. Her starched white coat made a crackling noise as it rubbed against her pant legs. Her office looked much the same as many others I'd seen, furnished with the same black metal desk, telephone, filing cabinet, and ergonomic office chairs. Blown by the breeze from the window, a tissue waved at me from another tissue box. Every room seemed supplied with them. Ms. Gordon walked over to her desk and pushed her black-rimmed glasses up on her nose as she lifted a pot of daffodils up to a spot on the window sill. She stopped to touch one of the flowers and smiled. It surprised me that in the light from the window her face looked so pretty.

"It's lovely to see spring flowers again, isn't it, Mrs. Evans?"

When I glanced up at the yellow daffodils on the sunny window sill, the room seemed to brighten. I nodded.

"Ellen told me you had some concerns about Ron's placement on the Brain Injury ward." She took a seat on the other side of the desk facing me.

"I thought he might improve faster around people his own age."

"Ron has a long way to go with his therapy. He's suffered severe head trauma as well as the spinal cord injury. I appreciate your concern about the age difference among patients. Please keep in mind, Mrs. Evans, he may not do as well as you think on the spinal ward. Some of our clients on the Brain Injury ward have spinal cord injuries as well."

But they're old! I thought. I'm not getting through to this woman. She doesn't understand how miserable life is for him there.

"Could you request a transfer for him at least? He's so unhappy where he is now."

"I believe the members of the team are aware of that," She consulted her file. "Ron is uncooperative at times. He has frequent outbursts of anger during his therapy sessions. Mood changes can be expected among some brain-injured clients. However, you understand our job is not to make your son happy but to prepare him for life outside the clinical setting. His head injury presents a major challenge."

I'm being stonewalled again, I thought, frustrated. I'd asked to see Ms. Gordon on Ron's behalf, to request a ward change for him. Instead she gave me a lecture. "I'm trying to understand, Ms. Gordon. I would like to see him have the chance to try. He knows the other boys. They get along so well. I don't know why…"

Ms. Gordon sighed. "I'll present your request to the team but I can't promise their decision will be any different. I'll call you back within the week and let you know if there's a chance he can be moved."

As I rose to leave, a single daffodil nodded its head in the breeze. Well that's more like it, I thought, leaving the room with at least a glimmer of hope.

As I walked out of the hospital I felt that our lives seemed to be nothing but a long journey on a road with many ups and downs, with many more ahead. I sighed. The pain in my gut, like a dark shadow of gloom, accompanied me wherever I went.

I had planned to go shopping on one of my days off. I got up early and dressed, gulped down my breakfast and put coffee in my thermos. I'd looked forward to a quiet morning stroll through the mall but before I could head out the door, the phone rang. "Mrs. Evans? It's Charlotte Gordon. Would you be able to come in today? I have some paper work for you to sign. I believe we have a new bed for Ron."

"Woohoo!" I hollered dropping the phone out of my hand onto the kitchen table.

"What's up?" asked Jeff, startled.

Ignoring him, I picked up the phone again. "I'll be there by ten o'clock, Ms. Gordon." I performed a little twirl around the kitchen. "Ron's being moved, Jeff. One of us has to go to the centre and sign something. Do you want to come along?"

"Uh, I promised George I'd go with him to the lumber yard. But if you need me…"

"No, that's okay. I told Ms. Gordon I'd be there by ten so it shouldn't be a long day."

Humming an old tune and smiling, I picked Ron's file up from the computer room. I gave Jeff a quick peck on the cheek, grabbed the car keys and flew out of the house. Susan, the occupational therapist, had provided Jeff with specifications for Ron's new living space in our house and he and George had been busy drawing up the plans. Even though it would be quite a while before Ron would be allowed to come home, Jeff wanted to get started pricing out materials for the project.

The file I had been keeping since Ron's accident had grown immensely. He had turned nineteen so more and more legal matters needed our attention. I assumed they had yet another paper to do with his care for me to sign. However, his possible move held far more importance for me than anything else.

I turned the steering wheel and swung into a parking stall in the family visiting area. I gave a quick wave to patients sitting outside enjoying the sun. As I hurried through the doors and into the foyer, Ellen looked up from her desk and called me over. "Hi, Mrs. Evans. The team is meeting in Room Five. You can go on down."

My previous visits, along with Ron's guided tours, had given me a good idea about the location of most of the meeting rooms. As I neared Room Five, Charlotte Gordon poked her head out and called, "Come on in. The team's finished its meeting."

Four people were in the room: The doctor in charge of Ron's case, a psychologist, a speech and language therapist, and Charlotte Gordon. They had little time for chit-chat but stopped long enough to introduce themselves. One by one, with the exception of Charlotte, they left the room, files tucked under their arms. I sat down and looked over at Ms. Gordon. I couldn't stop my heart from pounding.

She picked up the file on her desk and smiled. "We've looked at Ron's progress to date. There remain some valid concerns. However, the team has agreed to place him on the same ward as his former roommates."

I felt like jumping out of my chair and dancing around the room as tiny bubbles of excitement inside me rose to the surface. Charlotte continued, "Although they'll be on the same ward, individual schedules are different. His class times will not be the same as the others.

Ron is expected to continue with the Brain Injury program. He'll still see his roommates in the cafeteria and in the gym. Of course, they all have free time after dinner."

I could have hugged her. "I can't wait to see Ron's face. Thank-you for your help. I'll be sure to explain to him about attending his Brain Injury classes. I know how important they are to his recovery."

"I hope you do understand, Mrs. Evans. Your son's cognitive and language deficits are significant." Even though she looked at me with profound concern written across her features, she couldn't dampen my joy. I left the meeting room with a much different opinion of Ms. Gordon than I had when first we met. I realized she cared deeply about the recovery of each patient under her care. She had indicated in no uncertain terms that she expected patients and family members to work as diligently as the staff toward their rehabilitative goals.

Ron and his buddies had different schedules but met for meals in the cafeteria. Often they had therapy together in the gym. Visiting the gym turned out to be an eye-opener for me. One day Ron's therapist allowed me to watch as he taught Ron how to fall from his wheelchair to the floor and get up again without help. "Oh, no...," I gasped. Ron heard me, became distracted and fell with a thump onto the hard gymnasium floor.

"Mrs. Evans!" the instructor yelled. "If you can't be quiet, please leave."

I nodded my apology and sat down on one of the gym benches to watch the class. With his lower limbs paralyzed and his balance unstable, from his position on the floor Ron set the brake and put one hand up on the seat of the wheelchair behind him. He tried to push his body up from the floor and into the chair with the other hand. Beads of sweat shone on his forehead as over and over again he tried and failed.

He can't possibly be ready for this, my heart cried. Unable to watch any longer, I got up and ran out of the gym. I found an empty bench outside out of view, sat down and bawled like a baby. Ron survived the experience, of course. On my next visit I found him showing off to everyone who would stop and look his "falling and getting up" routine. "Kiece o' pake," he boasted in his chosen lingo of the day.

"I'm never sure what to expect next," I lamented to Jeff after a day at the centre. "You should see some of the guys racing up and down the halls doing wheelies. One of these days someone's going to get hurt."

Jeff snorted and slapped his knee. "Did you

hear yourself? They're already as hurt as they will ever be. Don't forget most of them are young like Ron, still feeling their oats."

Whenever Ron told me something, I didn't know if he was being truthful or not. Many times his language became so convoluted I couldn't understand him but the next day I felt positive he'd told me a group of them had signed up for a field trip to the mall where they would learn to ride the escalators while sitting in their wheelchairs. I envisioned them all tumbling headfirst down that steep moving staircase. When I asked the Recreation Director about it he laughed. "Yes, Mrs. Evans, we are going on a field trip to the mall but they won't be riding any escalators, not as long as I have anything to say about it. I think Ron got the message on the Memo Board mixed up. Take a look outside my door. You'll find the week's activities listed there."

I took time to look at the Memo Board. The field trip had been listed as he said. I found Ron's signature, an illegible scribble beside his name. I hadn't realized it before but the proof was right there. Ron had read the memo. He just had a distorted idea of its meaning.

Weary of the same old routine, on my next visit I decided to get a cup of coffee, go outside the cafeteria and watch Ron wheel around the garden walk. I sat on a bench to light a cigarette. The tobacco left a bitter taste in my mouth. I took a couple of quick puffs and butted out the cigarette, promising myself I'd quit soon. I glanced over at Ron again. With one eye still crossed he steered his shaky course around the walk. In a daring attempt to jump a high curb, he speeded up and flew out of his chair. Flat on his back in the gravel, he waved away my offer of help. With a pleased grin he got back into his chair without any trouble. "I metter cry turbs g'morrow," said he in his jabberwocky tongue.

Oh, Lord, I thought, I hope I'm ready for all this when "g'morrow"comes.

The day arrived soon after when I could take Ron to the mall for lunch. I imagined the lovely time ahead, strolling through the mall, stopping for lunch with him at a real restaurant. But our troubles began before we got into the car. One of the therapists showed me how to help him transfer into the vehicle.

"At first he'll have to use a transfer board. It won't take him long to learn how to keep his balance and transfer without the board. It's a matter of his safety at the beginning."

She showed me how to place the transfer board across from the seat of the chair to the seat of the car. No problem, I thought but because of his poor balance the board slipped and so did he. He held on, draped between the chair and the car. In the end, the therapist got under him and heaved him into the seat.

"He's still weak. As he gains strength he won't need the transfer board. He'll be able to do this by himself."

She showed me how to disassemble the wheelchair and load it into the trunk. It occurred to me I might benefit from some strength training myself. Off we went to the mall only to find the handicapped parking spot taken up by a sports car with no handicapped placard displayed. I pulled in beside the vehicle parked in the handicapped space but I had to open my passenger door wide enough to allow for the width of Ron's wheelchair. In the process of helping him into his chair, my door bumped into the other car.

"You scratched my car!" shouted a loud male voice.

I looked up to see a very fit young man run over to examine his side door panel. I lost my temper. "And you're parked in a handicapped space. If you're too dumb to read, there's a wheelchair symbol staring you in the face!"

For the first time, the man became aware of Ron in his wheelchair. "Uh, sorry. I just ran in for a few minutes. I wasn't gone that long."

Seething from my first encounter with such inconsiderate behaviour, I finished getting Ron into his chair and we headed for the mall entrance. I soon discovered that going out with him in public could be a harrowing experience. His wild, cross-eyed stare, screeching voice, sudden yelps, and frequent use of the F-word, attracted a lot of unpleasant attention. With his poor visual perception, he frequently wheeled into the path of others. I noticed most people were gracious in response to his obvious difficulties but some were not. I found myself feeling defensive and protective when I heard any criticism of my son's behaviour.

When Jeff and I visited Ron at the centre one day he showed his irritation with Ron's disruptive ways and rude language. He stood up, put on his cap and grabbed me by the arm. "Come on Jan. We're leaving." He turned to Ron. "I'm not staying here to listen to your foul language or put up with your rotten behaviour. It's unacceptable. Your mother and I will come back to visit when you decide to behave."

"Jeff," I pleaded when we reached the car, "he has a brain injury. We have to expect he'll act out at times. He can't help it."

Without a word, Jeff opened the car door and held it until I got in. He slammed the door shut, went around the other side, yanked the driver's door open and plunked himself behind the wheel. He turned to face me. "Don't make me say this twice. You're continually making excuses for the boy. He has to learn how to behave. Right now he's getting away with murder. Please don't talk about his brain injury. That's only part of it and you know it. Right now he's behaving like a manipulating little brat. Every time you accept that kind of behaviour you're telling him he can get away with it."

I didn't answer Jeff. There was nothing I could say to defend myself. I sensed there was something else, something darker than brain trauma causing Ron's changeable attitude and rotten manner. Another plague afflicted some of the centre's clients – street drugs. Vulnerable, seeking almost any remedy to ease their physical and emotional pain, some of the patients were easy prey for drug dealers who haunted the area. While the centre had a zero tolerance policy toward illicit drug use, still street drugs managed to get in.

Seated in the lobby one day my attention was drawn to a young man exiting the elevator. He moved in an awkward manner with one arm held out to keep his balance. I watched him as he stumbled toward the front door and wandered outside. A couple of men I suspected were not associated with the facility met him and took him behind some bushes out of sight of the security cameras. I sensed something amiss so I alerted the guard in the lobby. I learned later the boy had suffered a stroke as a result of cocaine use and the men I had seen him with in the bushes were there for one purpose, to supply him with more of the same.

TEN

Ron's speech had improved daily and his wayward eye straightened a little but his changeable moods and erratic behaviour continued to cause conflict. Sometimes he acted like the Ron we all knew and loved and sometimes not. No one could predict which Ron would emerge from one moment to the next. No longer did I look forward to spending time with him. When I visited I had to keep my guard up in case I said or did something to upset him. One sullen, sulky look or lengthy silence from him and my stomach did flip-flops. When obscenities erupted from his mouth my insides curled up in a tight ball of shame. I felt helpless to do anything but retreat, physically and emotionally. I noticed that the same behaviour happened in company with others. He manipulated social situations, using similar tactics. Often his coarse language brought conversation to a halt. When confronted about his poor conduct, he became teary-eyed and apologetic. He'd claim he couldn't remember what he had said or done. Everyone wanted to believe him because it was so out of character for him to act that way. His personality had undergone a distinct change. I looked to his brain injury for the reason.

Jeff and George had just finished the front ramp and proudly displayed their work to Susan, the occupational therapist from the rehabilitation centre. George had taken a liking to this willowy blond girl who spoke the language of building construction as well as any man. He grinned, opened the door and stepped aside as she entered the living room. Like two friendly puppies, he and Jeff led her in to see Ron's new bedroom and bathroom.

"This used to be our den," Jeff explained. "It was too small for this project so we removed a wall and expanded the room another three feet into the garage."

George chimed in, "We followed the specs you gave us. I think the bathroom turned out pretty well. Lots of room for his wheelchair now, eh?"

Susan's pretty blue eyes swept the room. She smiled at the two men as she pulled a measuring tape from her bag. "I'm so impressed with the ramp to the front door," she said, checking the bedroom and bathroom measurements. "This little suite is perfect."

"So you like the job we did?" asked George, expanding his broad chest even more than usual.

"Oh yes. Ron will have no trouble getting around. In fact, I'd say he's one lucky guy. Many of my clients don't have family or friends to support them or a home to go to when they're released from the centre."

Jeff looked down at his boots and choked up. "What happens to them?"

"They're referred to another agency. Subsidized housing for disabled adults is difficult to find. We hope to locate something suitable, perhaps a boarding situation. Although," she looked around at Ron's living area once more, "not many are as fortunate as Ron."

I hadn't thought about housing. I knew some of the centre's clients had no family near Drydon, but I hadn't stopped to consider they may not have a place to live. Since many were unemployable they would be dependent upon the government for funding and services.

When Jeff and I went to pick Ron up for his first home visit he met us in the foyer. "Hey Dad, Mom. Over here," he yelled.

Jeff winced at Ron's piercing voice, walked over to him and gave him a hug. "Hey, little buddy," he said. Slinging Ron's pack over his shoulder, Jeff walked beside him through the automatic doors of the centre. I toddled along behind, happy to have Jeff along to help Ron in and out of the car.

"Excited to see your new place, Ron?" I asked as we turned onto the highway.

"Yeah, wanna go home. Missy and Fluffy okay? Maybe they don't know me."

Jeff cautioned Ron. "This is your first home visit. Remember it's only for three days."

"Yeah. Hey, nice car dude," Ron screeched in his ear-splitting voice to a driver in the next lane. It's a wonder Jeff didn't swerve into oncoming traffic. Neither one of us had become used to Ron's sudden deafening screams. He seemed to have no clue his inappropriate comments to strangers might not always be welcome.

The weekend was filled with tension. Freed from the routine of the hospital, Ron went wild.

"Ron! Don't race your wheelchair around the house. You'll damage the walls."

"Can't help it, Mom. Doors not wide enough."

Jeff's stern voice rang through the house, "Take it easy, Ron. You're home on trial, remember? That means you're here to learn how to live in a home, not a big building. So listen to your mother. Don't crash into the walls."

Like a naughty little child, Ron hung his head and sank into his chair as a single tear ran down his cheek. "Okay, Dad. Sorry."

Ignoring his father's lecture of the previous day, Ron wheeled out of his bedroom door at top speed, leaving a deep gouge in the door frame as he passed through.

"Hey, Mom. Take Missy for walk, okay?"

Before I could answer he had pulled the leash down from its hook and waved it in front of the dog.

"Walk, Missy!" Tail wagging and tongue lolling out of her mouth, our collie allowed Ron to put the leash around her neck. Off they went, the frisky pup pulling her master's wheelchair down the front ramp. I hurried to the door and watched in horror as they raced along the sidewalk at breakneck speed. When one of Ron's wheels hit a crack in the concrete the chair turned over and they tumbled headlong into the neighbour's rose garden.

"Jeff! He's fallen into the rose bushes!"

Jeff came to the front door and took one look at Ron and Missy. "They got themselves into it and they can damned well get themselves out," he snorted.

"But Jeff, he can't reach his chair."

"Tough. He'll find a way."

My first instinct was to run and pick him up. Ron lay like a beached fish on the ground, howling with laughter. Somehow he and Missy managed to inch themselves out of their thorny landing place. Ron shifted himself along the ground until he reached the wheelchair then he flipped it upright and leapt from the ground into the seat. When he wheeled back into the house he still had a silly grin on his face. Missy followed, her head lowered, her leash dragging on the ground behind her and her tail between her legs. At least she had the sense to know that she'd done something wrong even if Ron hadn't.

I went and knocked on my neighbour's door. "I'm so sorry, Mr. Hansen. Ron and Missy had an accident and fell into your rose bushes. If any of them are damaged, I'll make sure they're replaced."

Mr. Hansen surveyed his garden bed. "No need, Janice," he said. "You've got your hands full with Ron, I can see that. I'll have a little talk with the boy when I see him then he might learn to keep his wheelchair on the sidewalk."

"Thanks, Mr. Hansen. You're very kind."

On Sunday morning I woke with a feeling of apprehension. *Something's happened to Ron.* I tossed back the covers, rolled out of bed and ran to his room. He sat upright in his bed, staring straight ahead. He gave no sign of recognition as I approached. The pupils of his brown eyes had grown large and black I watched with dread as he began to morph into his other self. Raging, cursing and screaming, he flung himself into his wheelchair and headed out the bedroom door. He seemed to be in a fit of some sort. In spite of his physical limitations his strength grew and he crashed his wheelchair into furniture, walls and anything else in his path.

"Jeff!" I screamed, attempting to grab hold of the wheelchair. By that time Ron had made his way into the kitchen. In his altered state we daren't let him out of the house.

My husband came running in, assessed the situation and without a word grabbed Ron from behind. He wrapped his arms around him and held on tight. Within a few minutes Ron's body relaxed. Slumped in his chair, he looked bewildered and began to cry, "Dad..."

Jeff and I looked at one another.

"What just happened here, Jan?"

"I don't know. He's had episodes before but never as bad as this."

I hurried to get a washcloth and towel from Ron's bathroom and, using warm water from the kitchen sink, wiped his sweat-covered face and neck.

"Ron," his father spoke in a sharp tone. "Ron, look at me. What's wrong?"

"Dad...Mom...scared."

I thought he'd had a nightmare. He had no memory of the incident and he didn't understand why we were so upset. I thought about the time, somewhere along his rocky road to recovery, being cautioned about the personality changes associated with head injury. I recalled flipping through the pages of our Brain Injury handbook and, deep in denial, dismissing those dreadful warnings.

Ron's weekend visits turned into trials for Jeff and me as well as for Ron. Throughout it all we discovered one irrefutable truth. When one member of the family becomes ill, the impact of that illness spreads throughout the family like a virulent disease.

Jeff phoned Kevin and filled him in about Ron's slow progress and his growing behaviour problems. Kevin flew in the next week for a family meeting.

"Okay," Jeff said. "I think we agree, if we're going to have the strength to cope with Ron we must first take care of ourselves. You've been trying to do too much, Jan. You're still trying too hard. So ease up a little, eh?"

"Yeah, Mom. No one expects you to do everything. You and Dad both need to take time for yourselves. Go see a movie once in a while. Heck, maybe you could even spend some time away together for a few days here and there, like you used to do."

"But Ron...," I butted in.

"Mom, you can get a sitter for Ron when he's home. You guys are retired now. You can afford to have someone come in and help out once in a while."

But a sitter? I had no idea how Ron would accept the idea of having a babysitter. "But we'd have to find someone who's trained...if he had another episode like the last one..."

"I have something I'd like to say about that Mom. I know he's had a head injury and most of his crazy behaviour can be put down to that. I also realize he has some serious nerve pain and he's on some pretty heavy medication but I think you need to consider that something else may be at work here."

Jeff twisted in his chair and said, "Kevin and I have talked about this Jan. There's something about Ron we haven't discussed."

"Something we haven't discussed? What do you mean? Jeff, you know I've looked everywhere for help."

Kevin stood up, cleared his throat and in his firm male voice, spit it out. "Mom, he's using drugs."

I gasped. Drugs? Ron? Never! "He's never been mixed up with anything like that, Kevin.

You must be mistaken."

Kevin and Jeff exchanged knowing glances and Kevin stomped into Ron's room. I listened in stunned silence as I heard him rummaging through his brother's dresser drawers. I glanced over at Jeff but his eyes avoided mine. We had always been firm about personal privacy and trust so Kevin's invasion into his brother's personal space was foreign to me. Red-faced, Kevin strode back into the family room and flung a handful of stuff onto the coffee table. "There! Take a look for yourself, Mom."

Dazed, I picked up the bits and pieces Kevin had taken from Ron's room. There in front of me lay cigarette rolling papers, tweezers, charred parts of plastic pens, an old-fashioned lighter and some plastic bags that gave off a familiar pungent odour, the same smell I had noticed on Ron's clothing recently yet, in my determination to not believe it, had dismissed.

"What's this…?" I mumbled, turning my head away.

"It's pot, Mom, and you know it. Come on, look at it. Grass, weed, marijuana, whatever you want to call it, he's smoking it and God only knows what else."

"Stupid, stupid kid! He's screwing his head up even more," Jeff exploded.

I couldn't take it in. A few minutes earlier

we'd been talking about going out to a movie, taking a holiday and with Kevin's announcement it had all turned sour.

"But how…where…?"

"The stuff gets into the centre all the time. The last time I visited Ron he was sitting outside with a couple of guys I didn't recognize. When they saw me coming they left in a hurry. I asked Ron who they were but he lied to me. He said they were friends of someone else on his ward but I've seen these types before. I think you know what I'm talking about Dad."

Jeff put his arm around me and sighed. "Well, he'll be coming home for good soon. I'm not sure we're prepared for this."

I knew Kevin felt heartsick. He had been the one person brave enough to expose Ron's drug use. Concerned for his brother as well as for Jeff and me, I knew he hated to be the one to bring such news to light. In the end we agreed on one thing. We must stay as healthy and strong as possible if we hoped to be of help to Ron. We realized taking care of this different and often unlovable Ron would not be an easy task.

For the first time since his accident I doubted the happy, carefree young man we once knew would ever come home again. Yet I clung to the notion that I must be the one to care for him as I had done during his childhood. I couldn't bear to face the fact that I would never be able to "kiss it and make it better". Ron had serious, multiple problems and so had I. In my efforts to find help for him I scrambled to consult a whole new set of experts in the fields of spinal cord and brain injury and then, drug addiction.

"His intellect is in the low to normal range. The area of Ron's brain affected is related to impulse control, memory, as well as reasoning and social skills. Socially and emotionally he functions somewhere between five and fourteen years of age. His behaviour, his social skills vacillate between those of a very young child and an adolescent. His poor short term memory could explain his bewilderment when he's faced with his unacceptable behaviour. He may not remember what he has done or said, or it may be he's learned to use that as an excuse, as some children do. While continued therapy may help, in my opinion it's doubtful he'll reach the potential for his age."

That statement, while not verbatim, is what I heard from one of the many experts who examined Ron. I still refused to accept that man's theory any more than I accepted that of the unknown doctor I'd met while Ron lay in a coma in the I.C.U. at Drydon Hospital.

Shortly after our meeting with Kevin, Ron came home. His drug use had been brought into the open. However, whenever Jeff and I tried to discuss the subject with him, he evaded the issue. His favourite avoidance technique would be to go into his room, sit in his chair or lie on his bed and sulk. This silent treatment appeared to be his most effective tactic whenever he wanted to avoid the topic of drug abuse.

Although now he lived at home full-time, Ron still went to the centre for outpatient therapy. At times, he would be picked up and delivered home by a volunteer driver. At other times, since Jeff's health had improved, he drove Ron to his appointments while I stayed at home.

"Ah, it's good to come home to a nice supper with my wee wife," Jeff would say as he nuzzled his whiskered chin into the back of my neck.

"Yuck! You two are so mushy," Ron complained with a knowing smirk on his face.

He'd been working on his language skills with the therapist and everyone noticed how much he had improved but other deficits remained such as his use of marijuana and, as Kevin had put it, "God only knows what else." The unknown "what else" concerned us more.

Jeff and I did not approve of most of the people with whom he associated. We suspected they were part of the drug scene. They were not welcome in our home but we knew Ron met them at coffee shops or hung out with them on the street. He had been seeing a drug counsellor but we had no idea how those sessions had progressed. Ron had turned nineteen and was legally an adult, so such files were confidential. Unless he had been declared incompetent, without his consent we could no longer access his personal information.

"Dave!" Ron greeted his Paraplegic Association counsellor one morning after Ron had moved home. David Hall had become a good friend and a frequent visitor to our house. He assisted Ron with his transition into the community. Dave, a quadriplegic, drove a van outfitted with a side lift that allowed him to get in and out of his vehicle without transferring from his wheelchair. Ron loved to talk to Dave about cars and especially about when he could apply to take his driver's exam.

"You're not ready to drive yet, Ron," I said, trying to steer their conversation away from that scary topic.

"Dave came over here to talk to me, not you," Ron cut in one day, his temper flaring. He turned his chair around and whipped into his room. Dave smiled then wheeled behind him into their private place where they could talk "man-talk".

I understood that motorists who suffered a brain injury could lose their license to drive for at least one year. However they could be eligible to apply for a new license after that time. Ron's year had long passed and without telling his dad or me he applied for his license.

At Drydon Rehabilitation Centre they had an instructor who taught those in wheelchairs how to operate vehicles equipped with hand controls. He decided if a client would be referred to take the Motor Vehicle exam. If so he'd make arrangements for an examiner to come to the centre to administer the required tests.

Following months of speech and language therapy, Ron spoke in a normal fashion and appeared fine, especially if he had reason to impress others. At home however, it was a different story. His short-term memory, spatial and visual perception and his judgement were, in my opinion, dismal. He either could not or chose not to control his impulsive ways and he often used offensive language. He made sure that none of that was obvious to those who mattered most when it came to getting his license.

"Hey Mom, Dad, come here. You won't believe what I got!"

Ron's driver had delivered him home from the centre. Jeff looked up as he entered the front door. "What's up, Ron?"

Ron wheeled into the kitchen waving a piece of paper in his hand.

"It's my license, Dad. I passed!"

I could have fainted. "Your license? Ron you don't have a car. I don't think you'll be driving any time soon."

"Yes I will. I had insurance, remember? I found out that's one of the benefits from my insurance settlement. They pay for a new car with hand controls to replace the one that got totalled and my wheelchair and medical aids are paid for, too. They have a legal counsellor at the centre and he helped me fill out all the papers. I'm going out tomorrow to look for a car."

I put my head down in my hands. Jeff and I had known about the settlement but hoped Ron wouldn't discover his insurance benefits included a new vehicle. Oh great, something else to worry about, I thought, shaking my head and turning away.

Soon after Ron bought his car, the telephone began to ring with complaints from the neighbours about his driving. We lived in a cul-de-sac and the parents with small children had become concerned when they saw him racing around the neighbourhood. Speeding tickets and fines mounted up. In short order, his nice new car had more body damage than any of us could have imagined possible yet neither Jeff nor I could do anything about it. We didn't have the right to take his keys from him. We couldn't take his license away. No matter what agency I phoned, I was reminded, "He is an adult, Mrs. Evans. As long as he pays his fines and keeps up his insurance, there is nothing we can do."

Knowing he had that prized and potentially deadly driver's license in his hands, our anxiety grew daily.

ELEVEN

A lovely, warm spring morning enticed me outside to work in the front garden. The moment I stepped outside, I heard Ron's terrible shrieking. The sound stabbed like a knife to the head.

"You oughta keep that kid locked up!" the neighbour on the opposite side of the road yelled. I brushed the hair from in front of my eyes and looked across the street. Ron sat in his wheelchair screaming as he watched our neighbour, old Mr. Mason, pull his remote-controlled truck out of the tulip bed, tear off its antenna and heave it across the yard. With wheels still spinning, the truck landed on its top, as useless as an upended turtle.

"You old fart!" Ron screamed at the man. "Mom, he wrecked my truck!"

I raced into the street, grabbed the back of Ron's wheelchair and gave it a mighty push toward our front door ramp. "You...," I spoke, gritting my teeth, "...get into the house right this minute." Ron rolled away fuming and swearing.

"I'm sorry, Mr. Mason," I apologized. "I

don't think Ron meant to run his truck into your tulip bed. If there's anything…"

Mr. Mason was in no mood for apologies. "That brat of yours is ruining the whole neighbourhood. You and your husband better do something. If he's not pulling a stunt like this one, its something else," he raged, shaking his limp tulips in my face. "He swears like a drunken sailor and drives that damned car of his like a maniac. And that's another thing," he raved on, his face red with anger. "He's a menace behind the wheel. I had to report him to the police twice this week."

It was only ten o'clock in the morning and already I felt exhausted. The sun beat down and beads of sweat formed on my forehead and trickled down my flushed cheeks. I couldn't think of anything else to say to the man so I simply shrugged and wandered back into the house. My gardening could wait for another day.

"What happened out there?" asked Jeff. "I heard a lot of yelling and Ron thumped into the house banging his wheels up and down. He's sure mad about something."

"Mr. Mason smashed his remote-controlled truck. Ron drove it over his driveway and knocked down his tulips. I don't think I can take much more of this. It's not just Mr. Mason. You know he gets cranky about everything but we have some lovely neighbours. The space between the houses is so small," I said, pushing my fingers through my hair, "that Ron's screaming and cursing disturbs everyone. I can't say I blame them. If we had young children who had to listen to that kind of language we'd be upset too."

"Yeah, George and I talked about that. It doesn't bother him but he lives alone so he just shuts the windows. The way Ron drives though, well...I'm concerned too, with all the little kids playing in the cul-de-sac. What are we supposed to do?"

Ron came out of his room. A footstool in the family room stood in his way. Cursing, he ran his wheelchair into it and tipped it over. "I'll get back at that old fart," he ranted. "I'll get my friends to come over here some night. They'll fix his damned tulips."

"Ron!" Jeff snapped. "I won't have that kind of talk in this house. Never, never threaten to harm anyone or anything, understand?"

"It's not fair," Ron moaned. "He smashed my truck. I could report him to the police."

I didn't know this crazy person. Ron had never acted or spoken that way before his accident. I had stopped blaming everything on his disabilities. His use of drugs, his choice of friends, played a large part in his continued clashes with the neighbours and with us.

I had discovered that he was an easy target for drug dealers. Not readily accepted among those his own age, he drifted toward people operating on the fringes of society. They accepted him as long as he had money. I noticed though, when halfway through the month Ron's money ran out, his new friends disappeared as well.

"Well, have you got any ideas?" I asked my husband one evening a few days later.

He turned his attention away from the hockey game. "Maybe we should look for a bigger place, somewhere further out in the country. It would give us room to breathe and get Ron away from these druggies. He's being dragged down more each day. It would do him good to get some distance from them. We could manage living in a rural area. After all, we don't have to commute to work anymore so we're pretty well free to live where we choose."

I understood what Jeff meant. Everything had gone wrong. Ron had slipped in so many ways. Although he had a closet full of good clothes, he chose to look grubby, wearing ripped jeans, his tee shirts riddled with cigarette burns. His identity had undergone a change for the worse, reflecting that of the members of his new social circle.

"Then that's what we'll do, Jeff. Let's give Murray a call."

Murray Campbell had helped with our other real estate transactions and we knew we could depend on him. Jeff made the call. Murray advised that we first drive around the different areas we might consider for a future home. So we went for long, lovely drives that led to many pretty, yet modern villages about the countryside. On one of our early evening excursions, we stopped for dinner at a restaurant overlooking a small rural town. Seated at a table by the window we enjoyed a panoramic view of the village. As dusk fell it transformed the scene below us as lights of the town centre twinkled in the changing light. One by one, farmhouses, cattle and horse barns, spaced far apart, shot their tiny sparks of light into the darkness. We walked out onto the restaurant terrace and breathed in the sweet smell of hay while we listened to a colony of frogs croaking their love songs into the night.

"This is it!" we exclaimed in unison.

Early the next day Jeff asked Murray if he would make arrangements for us to look at homes in our chosen area. My mind kept returning to the terrace of the restaurant and its lovely view and we asked Murray if he could find any listings nearby. My heart was set on that particular location and I didn't want to consider any other.

I had just started dusting the living room the next day when the phone rang. Leaving the dust cloth on the table, I hurried into the kitchen, "Hello. Oh, Murray, don't tell me you've found us a house already."

"I think I may have Jan. It's listed with another agent, but it's fairly large, on two acres right in the area you liked. Actually it's not too far from the restaurant you and Jeff mentioned."

"When can we see it? Jeff's gone out for an hour or so but we can go and have a look any time."

"Great. I'll call the other agent and we'll set up a time. It's empty except for a house sitter so it could be fairly soon. I'll call you back in about an hour."

When Jeff came in the door, I didn't give him time to put his packages down before I began to tell him my news. "Now don't get excited Jeff, but Murray called and he's found a place for sale right where we asked him to look. He's going to call back soon."

"Excited? Who's excited?" And he grabbed me around the waist and we twirled about the room. "We'll ask George to Ronny-sit. They get along okay. Ron doesn't usually try any of his stuff with George."

"We haven't got an appointment yet, silly. Wait until Murray calls."

"Okay. You know Jan, I've got a good feeling about this."

Jeff spotted the for-sale sign first. He swung the car onto the blacktopped driveway leading down to the house. On either side of the drive branches of huge cedar and fir trees bent to form a shady, green canopy. At the front of the large home the driveway widened into a circular parking area.

"My goodness, Jeff, there's room for at least a dozen cars."

Murray had reached the place ahead of us. He stood on the front steps and waited until we got out of our car. When we approached, he fished the keys out of his pocket and unlocked the door, stood aside and motioned us into an elegant foyer. We stepped up a few stairs into a spacious living room. Ceiling-high windows looked onto a wrap-around balcony and out toward the back of the property. From the living room we walked into a combined family room and kitchen. My heart skipped a beat when I saw the room of my dreams, a real country kitchen.

Murray didn't have to say a word as Jeff and

I ran from room to spacious room. The newly-renovated farmhouse boasted five thousand square feet of living comfort. We couldn't believe our good fortune when we went down the stairs from the kitchen to the lower level. A finished one-bedroom apartment appeared before us. Its large living room led out through sliding glass doors onto a concrete patio. From the patio, to our delight, we could see the sky-blue water of the in-ground swimming pool.

"What do you think, Jeff?" asked Murray, smiling.

"It's perfect. We'd have to do a little work on the downstairs bathroom and build ramps so Ron can get into the main house, but think, Jan...," Jeff turned to me, "...if we decide this is the property we want, Ron will have a place of his own and so will we."

We made our move at the beginning of summer. I couldn't wait to lower my tired body into the lovely pool, to float around on my air mattress with a nice cold drink in my hand and gaze up at the wispy, white clouds as they drifted across the sky. I thought, if I'm in heaven then our cat, Fluffy, and dog Missy, will have found an animal paradise.

Once we settled in we discovered we had moles in residence in the yard. Our cat, Fluffy, being a natural hunter took advantage of the opportunity to hone her hunting skills. Each morning we found evidence of her night's adventure as we picked up and disposed of her kill but the moles proved to be quick learners and soon moved on to a habitat more suited to their survival.

"Mom! Come and see what I found. It's a baby rabbit!"

Jeff and I got up from our lounge chairs on the balcony and looked down. Ron had a little rabbit in his arms. "You'll have to take it back to its nest, Ron," said Jeff. "That's a wild rabbit. If you found the nest then Missy and the cat will find it, too."

"Oh no, what'll I do? I don't want Missy to kill it."

"Just a minute, Ron," I yelled. I found an old laundry basket and threw it down to him. "You'll need to cover the nest with the basket but first make a hole near the top of the basket, and then turn it upside down over the nest. That way the mother rabbit can get in and out and the babies will be safe."

Jeff yawned and stretched, "I'll go down and help him. He can't hold the rabbit and do all that at the same time. Where did you learn so much about wild life?"

I smiled and tried not to look smug as I sat and gazed out over our immense back yard.

The part of our property not covered in old-growth trees and wildflowers had been planted in grass. Since Jeff's doctor didn't want him to do any heavy work, someone else would have to maintain the grounds. To my surprise, I came up with an answer to the problem. Before his accident, Ron had done some work for a landscaping company and he'd always enjoyed working outdoors. I'll have a talk with Jeff, I thought, closing my eyes.

"Jeff, would you like to go shopping with me?" I asked later.

"Shopping? You've got to be kidding. You know I hate sitting on those hard benches in the mall waiting for you to finish your shopping."

"Not that kind of shopping. I want to go to that tractor place on the highway."

"I knew the country air would have an effect on you but I didn't think you'd end up wanting to buy a tractor."

"Well, not exactly a tractor. I am thinking about a ride-on lawn mower. They make them with hand controls. If we had that kind of a mower Ron could cut the grass."

"Yeah, I suppose he could. The kid across the street asked me if we had any work for him. Ron won't be able to empty the grass cuttings but if we got the other boy to help, it could work out."

The next day we drove to visit the tractor lot. We found a used ride-on lawn mower with hand controls, exactly the one we had in mind. When the delivery man unloaded the equipment Ron leapt out of his wheelchair into the mower seat and started the motor. I thought I saw tears in Jeff's eyes as he watched his son drive the mower around the grassy back field. That Saturday our young neighbour, Connor, came over and helped with the edging and emptied the mower bag. Ron made it clear from the beginning that he was in charge of the operation. Within a short time our elderly neighbour next door benefitted from Ron's new occupation as weekly, sitting like a king on his noisy mobile throne, he scooted over to mow her grass.

"Hey Ron, hand me the crescent wrench," I heard a gruff male voice say one afternoon. I peered over the balcony railing to see a strange man dressed in grease-covered striped overalls bending over the engine of our lawn mower.

"Here you are, Jim," said Ron, handing the man a wrench. Ron glanced up at me, "Hey Mom, this is Jim. He lives down the road."

The man lifted his head from the mower engine, "Hi there, Mrs. Evans. Young Ron here needed a little help. Nothing serious though. I'll have it fixed in a jiffy."

"Jim's a heavy duty mechanic, Mom."

A heavy duty mechanic? The man looked like an angel to me. Ron loved mechanics. I thought of the many times he had "fixed" his toy cars by taking them apart so he could put them back together. In fact he would take apart and examine anything with wires and wheels, including my household appliances. I used to haunt thrift stores for used clocks and radios so he could take them apart – anything to keep his little fingers away from my kitchen tools.

"It's nice to meet you, Jim. Would you like a coffee?"

"No thanks. Gotta go home and muck out the horse stall."

During that summer Ron and Jim spent many happy hours working together, either on mower maintenance or under the hood of Ron's car. Except for the nerve pain in his legs, Ron seemed fairly healthy. Strong and wiry, he could manage many jobs requiring physical strength. What caused him the most difficulty were jobs that called for abstract reasoning and good judgment. That and his impulsivity kept getting in the way of his success with work-related activities. He frequently became frustrated when we tried to reason with him. As a result of his brain injury he had great difficulty thinking a problem through in a logical way. His one try at volunteer work failed. Because of his ongoing pain and changeable moods we couldn't tell from one day to the next if he'd be able to get out of bed, let alone work. Jeff and I were also aware that Ron's use of marijuana as a recreational drug could turn into full-blown drug dependence. The dark spectre of drug addiction seemed to hover over our son, waiting to lay claim to his soul.

We didn't know what to do for him as his blue moods deepened but help came from an unexpected source. A phone call from his cousin, Jordan, improved his outlook. Jeff's brother, Andrew, owned a farm machinery business in the next province and the family offered Ron an opportunity to work in their office and sometimes on their cattle ranch. Ron jumped for joy in his chair when he received the phone call and couldn't wait to tell us all about it. I wanted to rejoice with him but couldn't shake the bad feeling I had about the idea from the beginning.

"Now wait a minute, Ron. It's kind of Uncle Andy to offer but I don't think you're ready to leave home just yet. You can be a handful at times. I don't believe Jordan understands how difficult working at a steady job could be for you. You'd have to live on your own if you're working in town. I don't think you're ready for such a big step. What do you think, Jeff?"

"I'm not sure. I'll phone Andy and we'll talk it over."

Our lovely summer had turned into fall and I knew that Ron had never experienced the frigid temperatures of a prairie winter. All he knew about cattle ranching was the bits he had picked up from his visits with his cousins during his summer holidays.

"Mom, I'll be okay. Why not let me go for a while? If it doesn't work out I can always come home again," Ron begged.

"I've spoken with Andy. He thinks the change might do Ron some good," Jeff said later. "He says Ron can drive one of the ATVs whenever he's at the ranch and transit around town is excellent. It might be a good experience for him."

Outnumbered, I gave in and we prepared Ron for his Wild West adventure. I hoped Jeff's relatives had some idea of the experience they were in for.

The morning of Ron's flight Jeff didn't feel well so I took our son to the airport. We drove through the dense morning fog customary for the season. Ron sat beside me in the passenger seat, his flight documents clutched in his hand. A quick glance at his fingers revealed nails bitten down to the quick.

He must be terrified, I thought, not far off that state myself.

Through the grey mist the sprawling airport terminal loomed before us. His flight could have been cancelled because of the weather, I thought as I wound through the approach to the airport. On one hand I hoped the fog would lift. On the other, I would have welcomed any excuse to turn the car around and drive him back home.

Ron stuck his head out the car window. "Straight ahead, Mom," he said. "I can see the handicapped sign. Someone's pulling out so we can park in front."

I relaxed my tight grip on the steering wheel and slipped into the convenient parking spot.

After pulling Ron's wheelchair from the trunk I attached the wheels and pushed it to the passenger side of the car. Ron hopped into his chair and wheeled to the back of the car to help me load his baggage into a cart. When we entered the terminal the airport schedule board displayed its stark message. The plane would leave on time.

The night before at his farewell dinner, Ron had surprised us all with a new shorter hair style. That morning, dressed in cool designer jeans and jacket and wearing his western hat, he wheeled through the cavernous building with an air of confidence I suspected he didn't feel. He stared straight ahead, as if looking forward to a fresh start in a new city.

Ron's brief goodbye showed a sign of his new-found independence. After he checked in he allowed me to give him a hasty kiss on the cheek before he wheeled toward the boarding area.

"'Bye, Mom. Take care of Dad and Missy and Fluffy."

I followed him as far as the barrier and a stern security officer would allow. In the distance, I could see the special chair used to carry him on board. His fellow passengers brushed past me, moved in behind his wheelchair and blocked my view. I stood on tiptoe and watched as he disappeared into the crowd.

Waiting and watching with friends and relatives of other passengers on the flight, I leaned against the airport window until the plane took off then jostled along by the departing crowd, I left the building and headed to the car.

The smog outside stung my eyes. Blinking, I unlocked the door and fell in behind the wheel. The painful lump that had sat in my stomach all morning rose to the surface. Sobs, held back since the night before, broke through an emotional dam. Before I could put my key in the ignition, they erupted in a flood of tissue-defying tears. I slumped down into the seat in a quivering, convulsing heap. After a while I pulled myself together then I started the engine and drove away from the airport. By the time I reached the highway, the sky had cleared to a brilliant blue but my own fog held me in its gentle mist, softening the harsh reality of the day.

When I reached the house I tried to concentrate on my plans for the rest of the day. I climbed the few steps to the kitchen then stopped on the landing. As if drawn by a magnet I moved toward the door leading down to my son's apartment. I flicked the light switch at the top of the stairs and my fingers passed over a tattered Tasmanian Devil decal still clinging to the switch plate. The rooms filled with light revealing a familiar disorder. Robot-like, I began to tidy the place. Ron's castoff clothing sat in piles on the floor. If he'd been there, I would have reminded him of his messy ways. Instead, I bent down to pick up a damp towel he'd dropped and discovered it still held his scent.

Ron's pleading voice rang in my ears, "Please understand, Mom. I want to go. It's the chance I've been waiting for, to get some training and do something with my life."

But who will take care of him when he needs help? Have I packed enough warm clothing for him? Thoughts of impending disaster ran through my mind.

It looked like a tornado had touched down in his apartment. I tried to bring some order to the place but gave up. Plopping myself down into his brown overstuffed chair, I brushed without effect at the cat hairs embedded in the material. Fluffy hopped up on the arm of the chair and purring, rubbed her face against my shoulder. How he loves his cat, I thought. I sneezed and put her down on the floor then got up from the chair. She mewed, winding in and out of my legs as I put her food and water out. At the same time, I heard our dog, Missy, barking and whining outside. When I saw her pawing at the glass of the sliding door, I went and let her in. The animals are going to miss him, too.

Autumn turned into winter and Jeff's health deteriorated so that he could no longer manage to climb stairs or putter in the garden. He used to enjoy wandering about the property or going for walks through the surrounding hills but he had begun to notice a familiar shortness of breath. Twice he'd fallen and hurt himself so badly that he had ended up in the hospital. It became clear we would have to find a smaller one-storey house if we hoped to accommodate his mobility needs. Once again, Murray came to our rescue and with Kevin's help we moved to a smaller home near the town centre. Jeff improved somewhat after that but I missed my larger home.

"Hi Mom. I'm doing fine," Ron reported when he phoned home. "I'm still in the apartment Jordan found for me. It's close to town. They built a ramp for me at work so it's easy getting into the office. I'm putting data into the computer. How's Dad?"

I told Ron all the news but something in his voice concerned me so I gave Jordan a call. "I have the feeling Ron's not telling me everything, Jordan. I know he doesn't like me to interfere but I wondered if you had any concerns."

"As a matter of fact, Auntie Jan, we've been having problems with Ron. Everyone here likes him but often he makes rude remarks, embarrassing the girls. You understand we can't ignore that kind of thing. He's not dressing properly for the office either and he's been showing up to work late. I know he's in a lot of pain but I think some of his problems might have to do with the people he's been hanging around with lately." My heart sank.

After I'd discussed the call with Jeff, I called

Jordan back. Supportive of Ron as ever, his cousin felt bad he had to deliver such news but I understood that Ron's behaviour, memory lapses and lack of judgment, as well as his outbursts of temper, made his life and the lives of those working with him, extremely difficult. When Ron next phoned home, I tried to pin him down, "Ron, if you can't manage to work on a steady basis; it's okay. Maybe you tried to take on too much at once. No one expects you to work if you're not well."

He began to sob over the phone. "I try, Mom. But they don't understand. It's because I'm in a wheelchair. Everyone thinks I'm some kind of freak."

Familiar with the people Ron worked with, I suspected what Ron told me wasn't the entire story. I knew his cousins tried their best to include him in family gatherings and his fellow workers wanted him to succeed. Whether he believed what he told me or not, didn't matter. In the end, Ron couldn't live up to his own unrealistic expectations. In pain and confusion much of the time, his work performance and health declined and I believed that, from what I learned from Jordan, drugs had entered the picture once more.

One day, the call came from Ron. "Mom, Dad, I need to come home."

TWELVE

At least his timing was good. By now it was early July and Jeff and I had planned to drive to the prairies for the city's annual rodeo so bringing Ron back home with us wouldn't be a problem. We had always enjoyed the drive from the coast through the mountain passes and past green glacier lakes. I found on the long drive that whenever Jeff took the wheel I relaxed and had trouble keeping my eyes open. On the last leg of our journey, I think I slept most of the way.

Knowing how difficult it could be finding accommodations during rodeo week, we'd booked our hotel room well in advance. As soon as we registered, we showered and changed into our jeans and western shirts then I called Ron. "We just arrived at the hotel. Would you like to go out for dinner?"

"Sure Mom. I'm all dressed. I figured you'd be getting in soon."

Jeff took the phone out of my hand. "Ron! I've got your address and if you're ready we'll pick you up in about half an hour, okay?"

"Okay Dad. I'll be waiting at the entrance.

It's the big blue and white building. You can't miss it."

I saw his wheelchair first. Ron sat hunched down in the seat, a cowboy hat hiding his face. His arms were crossed and his long legs dangled awkwardly from the chair. Tipping his hat back, he squinted into the afternoon sun, eyes fixed upon the road. As we approached the entrance, I could see he didn't look well. Dark shadows ringed his eyes and his face had a jaundiced look. When he spotted our car he straightened up and, wheeling with all his might, raced toward the edge of the road.

"Mom, Dad!"

Jeff pulled up to the curb and switched off the engine. Both of us jumped out of the car at the same time. Ron lifted up his arms and wrapped them around our legs in a fierce grip. And then his face crumpled and his body heaved as he broke down and wept.

Jeff wiped the tears from Ron's cheeks then handed him the soggy handkerchief to blow his nose. "It's all right, Ron. We'll sort things out as we go along."

"There's plenty of time," I joined in, running my hands through his hair.

"I'm sorry Mom. I couldn't explain over the phone. I messed up. I got so screwed up I didn't know what to do. I let everybody down.

They're all going to hate me."

Jeff pushed his Stetson back on his head and put his hand on Ron's shoulder. "Nobody hates you, Ron. Now, there's a fine steak dinner waiting for us, so whadda ya say we saddle up and put on the old feed bag, eh, little buddy?" he drawled, doing his movie cowboy imitation.

Ron and I both groaned then turned away and snickered.

"I started to pack, Mom but there are still clothes in the dryer. I haven't finished the bills and stuff. Could you guys come over tomorrow and give me a hand?"

Jeff opened the car door and Ron hopped in the front seat while I took the wheelchair apart and shoved it into the trunk.

"We'll talk about that tomorrow," I said. "Uncle Andy expects us to visit them at the ranch and we've got tickets for the rodeo. So let's wait and see how the week goes."

"All right, Mom, but you haven't seen my apartment yet."

"That's okay. I can imagine the state of your apartment," I replied with more than a hint of sarcasm. I settled down in the back seat as Jeff started the car and we headed for the restaurant.

Lively country music played and got my

toes tapping. City-born, I couldn't help but be swept up in the spirit of rodeo week. I wanted to leap out of my seat, grab my husband and join in the line dancing. Jeff, a country boy through and through, made himself right at home. Glancing over at Ron, I noticed him grinning across the table at us. His face brightened as he too became caught up in the festive atmosphere of the restaurant. Everyone wore cowboy hats, at least most of the people we met did. The city crawled with tourists like us and western wear was de rigueur for the week.

A pretty waitress dressed in a studded jean skirt and jacket, skipped over in her cowgirl boots to deliver our steaks and caught Ron's roving eye. By the time we left the restaurant the temperature had dropped and the sun had set. When we reached Ron's apartment, I shivered as I waited for Jeff to take his wheelchair from the trunk. With Ron back in his chair, I bent down to kiss him goodnight.

"See you tomorrow, son. We'll be over about eight o'clock to check out the apartment, so get an early night."

"Thanks Mom, and thanks for the dinner, Dad. I had a great time."

Jeff and I drove back to our hotel and, although we should have been exhausted from our long drive and late dinner, we both felt a certain energy that seemed second nature to the local people. Must be something in the water, I thought.

We needn't have brought the alarm clock with us. Spot on six o'clock the next morning we were both wide awake. Jeff took his turn in the shower while I phoned the hotel desk and ordered our morning coffee. Jeff came out of the shower wearing nothing but the bath towel he'd wrapped around his waist. He strolled over to the balcony doors and pulled open the blinds. The bright prairie sun shone down, lighting up the room. If we hadn't already been awake by then that strong sunlight would have persuaded us to get up and get going.

Jeff seemed happy as he rummaged through his bag to find the perfect outfit for the day. Slim-fitting denim jeans still sat well on his lanky body. A huge silver horseshoe belt buckle glistened at his waist as he strutted about the room in his heeled western boots.

He still looks pretty good to me, I thought with a smile.

We heard a light tap on the door and Jeff opened it to a slight young man in western garb carrying our coffee tray.

"Would you set it out on the balcony table please?"

"Yes, ma'am," he answered and walked out

to the balcony to put the coffee things on the table. Jeff walked back with him to the door and fished in his wallet for a tip.

"Call down to the desk if you need anything else folks," he said as he left the room.

We sat out on the balcony and savoured our first coffee of the day. An early morning chill hung in the air but oddly enough it didn't seem to bother us. With a groan, Jeff slapped his stomach, got up from his chair and carrying his coffee cup into the room, picked up the phone and called Ron.

"Hi, Ron. I thought you'd like to have breakfast with us. If you're up and dressed, we can be there in fifteen minutes."

"Did you get him out of bed, Jeff?" I asked after Jeff hung up the phone.

"Nah, he's excited we're here and raring to go. After breakfast we can go back to his place and see what needs doing."

Our breakfasts were huge. The men ordered their usual eggs over easy with everything which included pancakes, bacon and sausages and all the hash-browned potatoes they could eat, all washed down with tall glasses of full-fat milk. I settled for a couple of poached eggs. When I looked around I noticed quite a few customers scoffing down big steaks along with their morning eggs. I couldn't understand how these people could take in all that food and still stay slim. It must be something in the water, I mused again and wondered if there was a way to ship this miracle elixir back to the coast.

Ron tucked into his meal like a starving man. He chattered on and on as he chowed down. He seemed relaxed and happy to be sitting at the table enjoying a family meal. After breakfast we drove to his apartment. I took one look around and called Jordan.

"Hello Jordy. We're at Ron's apartment and it needs a thorough cleaning before the owners inspect it. Do you know of anyone we can hire on short notice to do the job?"

"I'm way ahead of you, Auntie Jan. We have this guy, Jimmy, who does the office cleaning at night and he's always looking for extra day work. I have a duplicate key to Ron's place so I'll give it to Jim and send him over to do the cleaning while Ron's out with you."

With that taken care of, we made the rounds of town, enjoyed the hospitality of relatives and took photos of babies born since our last visit. We spent a couple of thrilling days at the rodeo and on our last day, wandered around the famous Heritage Village on the outskirts of town. We rode on the old diesel train and stuck our noses into fascinating historical shops set at the back of the raised plank sidewalks. Grabbing some food, we found a big picnic table outdoors and sat down to stuff ourselves. Our whole week was fun-filled and happy but by the end of the week we were all ready to head for home.

On one of our visits to the ranch, Jeff, his brother Andy and I had a long talk about Ron. Andy and his family had tried in every way they could to expose Ron to different areas of work but he didn't seem to fit in anywhere. Computer work gave him a headache and other office jobs that called for attention to detail ended up in confusion. His physical limitations excluded him from many jobs on the ranch. The one place where he succeeded was in their machine and electrical shop.

"That boy has a knack for mechanics," said Andy. "He did fine whenever we asked him to help out with the tractors or other machines but he's sure got a mouth on him and a quick temper too. He could put an old hand like me to shame in a cussing contest."

I cringed. I knew what Andy was talking about. If Ron couldn't manage to keep his bad manners in check within the accepting, yet rough and tumble environment of his uncle's ranch then I hated to think how he'd manage once he returned home.

Andy continued, "You know we all love

Ronny. I'm only sorry things didn't work out for him here. I've told him, and you make sure he understands, he's welcome to come back for a holiday next summer. We'll show him a good time." Jeff's big brother drew his oversized handkerchief from his pocket and blew his nose.

On the way home we tried to prepare Ron for the fact he wouldn't be living at home with us. We didn't have the room he needed in our small house and I knew Jeff couldn't take the upheaval living with Ron would bring.

Before we'd left home, we leased and furnished a nice one-bedroom suite for Ron in an apartment complex near our house. He would be independent but we would be nearby to help him if he needed anything. The main room of his unit opened out onto a shady garden patio, so not only could he wheel outside whenever he chose but he had a private smoking area as well.

When we took the elevator up from the underground parking area, Ron hung on to his duffel bag while Jeff and I carried the last couple of boxes of linens to the apartment. Jeff took the keys from his pocket and handed them to Ron who grinned, unlocked his door and wheeled into the main room. His bulging duffel bag landed on the floor and Jeff dropped the boxes down beside it.

"Hey, this place is all right, Dad. Did you notice the bus stop at the front entrance?"

"It's very nice. You'll find everything's handy and you can shop at the grocery stores down the street. Just keep in mind Ron, there are strict rules to follow. I'm leaving you a copy of the lease agreement to read over. It's important to be considerate of your neighbours. Please don't give your new address or phone number to strangers. The apartment is for your use. No one else stays overnight, understood?

"Ah, Dad. You don't have to tell me…"

"Yes he does, Ron," I interjected. "We realize you may feel lonely at times but we also know you have a tendency to get mixed up with the wrong crowd and that can lead to trouble."

"But what if they're my friends?"

"Ron," Jeff's voice sounded stern. "Remember the kind of friends you used to have. You know what we're talking about. You'll be comfortable here but you're a grown man and we can't watch over you all the time. Your mother and I want you to act in a responsible way, that's all."

"Yeah, I guess I understand. I'm sorry. But it's going to be hard, starting over again."

Ron had no idea how hard it would be to

make a new start. He had no personal source of income except for a disability pension of six hundred and fifty dollars a month. To be financially independent, it would be necessary for him to turn to a government agency for assistance.

"I can't fill out these forms, Mom," he told me one day when I dropped in for a visit. "I don't understand what they want."

"Ron, take it one question at a time and answer as truthfully as you can."

To complete and deliver the forms necessary to receive financial assistance would have been a challenge for most of us but for Ron, being put through bureaucratic "hoops" turned out to be another obstacle that put a strain upon his thought processes and fragile ego. In the end, his patient and overworked case manager helped him with the paperwork. She issued him a small cheque on an emergency basis. After that he obtained his permanent disability status and had his pension supplemented by an allowance of three hundred and fifty dollars. It sank in. Ron must learn to live on the princely sum of one thousand dollars a month.

Jeff and I helped him as much as we could, or rather, as much as Ron would allow. He became upset if we interfered too much, especially if it happened to be me doing the interfering.

"This is my place, you know," he raged at me one day when I stopped by. "Why don't you leave me alone? You hate my friends and you don't like the way I live my life, so why don't you just get out?"

On the advice of Ron's social worker, even though it hurt us terribly, that's what Jeff and I decided we must do. It didn't take long until he spiralled into depression. Whenever he visited our home he looked unkempt, unwashed and unhealthy. When other family members tried to talk to him, he became defensive and angry. As he pushed his family and concerned friends further and further away, he ignored Jeff's advice about the apartment rules and began to invite people of dubious character to stay with him. He began to view Jeff and me as the enemy.

"You two get out of my life! You don't want me around anyway. Look at me. I'm a useless cripple. The pain in my leg is so bad I can't get out of bed most days. And the doctor won't give me any more medication."

All this reminded me of the warnings of educators in the field of brain injury. The one most common was that brain-injured people may turn against those closest to them. Although Jeff and I tried to understand, we found it difficult to accept when our son's anger and frustration came our way.

"He can't go on like this, Jan. He has no money most of the time and he goes around town looking like a bum. He can't manage on his own much longer."

Never in my most frightening dreams did I expect to find any one of my children living under such horrific conditions. What used to be Ron's neat, respectable apartment became a place for street people to squat. The smell of marijuana and, as Kevin would say, "…God only knows what else," permeated the place. Cigarette burns appeared in the carpets and furniture. Anything of value soon disappeared.

"Ron! What happened to your television set? I bought it last week and now it's gone."

"I don't want to talk about it, okay?" he sulked.

"We had better talk about it. I can't keep spending money on things that go missing within a day or two. When I looked in your closet I couldn't find your new jeans. What's going on?"

"Okay Mom. So I got robbed. There, now you know. A couple of guys came in and took my T.V."

"Come on, Ron. Don't give me that story. With the security in this building, no one gets in the front door unless a resident buzzes them in. You must have let those people in yourself."

"I had to Mom. You don't get it, do you? Those guys had me outside with a knife at my throat. If I hadn't let them in they'd have killed me."

We had already received letters of complaint from the owner about unsavoury looking characters seen going in and out of Ron's apartment. Since Jeff and I had signed the lease, we were expected to deal with the problem or Ron would be evicted. He had nowhere to go. In addition to that, I discovered his new "friends" had introduced him to a cheque-cashing store. Ron told me he had been threatened and forced to write post-dated cheques on his account. When he presented the cheque at the cheque-cashing establishment, the funds would be advanced to him. Ron would hand the money over to his friends to purchase drugs. Not only did his money vanish before he received it but the store charged him exorbitant interest for their service.

"Okay, Ron," I said. "If you won't take care of the situation then I will."

"Mom, don't do anything, please. They'll know I told you and they'll kill me."

"Nobody's going to kill you. I'll go to the store and tell them not to cash your cheques and that will be that."

Of course, it wasn't that simple. When I visited the store and asked them to stop the practice I heard the now-familiar argument. "He's an adult, Mrs. Evans. We can't refuse to cash his cheques as long as he can prove he has an income."

I glared through the barred window at the clerk and assured her that indeed, I would see to it her store no longer cashed Ron's cheques. Armed with a letter from his doctor confirming his brain injury, as well as one from his government case worker, I had the account "red flagged". With that problem behind me, I began to breathe easier, though not for long.

Soon an infamous credit card ploy revealed itself. Before long, Ron's associates helped him apply for a credit card and without my knowledge he received that precious piece of plastic.

On one of my rare visits to him, I found a demand letter from a credit card company for immediate payment of an overdue account in the amount of five thousand dollars. I knew Ron hadn't purchased anything for himself, so I questioned him about the debt.

"I don't know, Mom. I don't even have the card. This guy took it."

"All right, Ron. Who is this guy and where does he live?"

"I don't know. He came and took it after it came in the mail. I don't know where he lives."

"Ron, did you give him your access code?"

"What's an access…oh, his girlfriend did that for me. I couldn't remember it anyway."

I didn't see any point in questioning him further. Ron had allowed his friends to do it to him again. In a fit of righteous anger, I phoned the credit card company to protest the practice of giving unlimited credit to a disabled person living on government assistance. The gentleman on the other end of the line informed me that as long as they had Ron's address and his social insurance number, they would issue a credit card in his name. When I asked an advisor at my bank about it, he said that what I'd been told by the company's representative had, unfortunately, been absolutely true.

There ought to be a law! I fumed.

The one bright spot in all of this came when Ron lost his driver's license. After one too many charges of impaired driving and fines he couldn't pay, a wise judge decided to take his license away. Jeff and I both breathed sighs of relief.

I had learned something along the way about enabling an addicted person. Kevin had warned me about that and I didn't want to help Ron in any way that would further his addictions. At the same time, I felt I must consider his medical needs and hesitated to remove his safety net altogether. He had turned away from so many positive influences in his life, I found it difficult to stand by and do nothing to help him.

"Hey, Mom. I haven't got any milk or eggs. Could you meet me downtown and give me ten bucks?"

"That's all right, Ron. I'll pick the groceries up for you and bring them over."

Bang! I heard his phone hit the floor. "Hello? Are you still there, Ron?" Then came a click and the line went dead but I continued to buy him food and once in a while, clothing. Even that turned out badly when a new jacket I had purchased for him went missing from his closet. As I tried to distance myself from his day to day life, I refused to give up hope. I knew there must be other parents out there who found themselves in the same heart-wrenching position.

"We have to let him go, Jan," Jeff said to me one day. "We have no control over him. Anyway, he's the one doing the controlling, or hadn't you noticed? I've listened to the way he talks to you. He screams at you to leave him alone and then he turns around and says he loves you. You get sucked in every time. Face the facts, honey. He loves his drugs more than he loves you, me or anyone else."

I heard the words but I didn't want to believe them. I hated Jeff for saying such awful things to me and I hated that he would even consider giving up on our son. In the end, because of his less-than-desirable roommates, Ron had to be evicted from his apartment. In the middle of a harsh winter he found himself on the streets without proper food or clothing. I found he slept in a homeless shelter from eleven at night until seven in the morning and was then turned out to fend for himself during the day.

Dependent upon his wheelchair, he was an easy target. We learned that every cent he received on pension day had been withdrawn from his account. It had been easy for wilier people than he to convince him to withdraw cash from the account. Another favourite trick was to deposit one of his cheques to a zero balance account in a bank machine and then immediately withdraw cash in the same amount. The practice of course, constituted fraud but offered these people another quick and easy way to obtain cash while leaving Ron to deal with the consequences. I couldn't convince him that taking money in that way could result in his being charged with theft.

"But I wrote a cheque," he'd explain.

"Ron, you can't cash a cheque when you know there's no money in your account. That's a criminal offence."

"But the bank gave me the chequebook, Mom."

I threw up my hands, trotted down to see my understanding bank manager and had the matter straightened out.

Street people stole his shoes and warm clothing while he slept. He ended up being admitted to Valleyview Hospital, seriously ill but as soon as he recovered he was released back onto the street. Because of his frail medical condition, the Valleyview Hospital doors continued to revolve as he contracted one antibiotic-resistant infection after another.

He began going around shoeless. Often he would appear at my door with nothing but hospital socks on his feet. When I asked him about it he told me his feet were swollen and he couldn't get his shoes on anymore. However, during one of his rare visits in between hospital admissions, I noticed blood dripping from one of his legs. When I asked him about it, he told me he had banged his leg against a metal door frame somewhere. When I bent down to examine his swollen foot, I smelled the unmistakable odour of rotting flesh.

Against his wishes, I tossed him into the car and drove him to see our family doctor. He had him admitted to Ogden Hospital that day. Ron had developed pressure sores on his calf and ankle and left unattended, the wounds had become badly infected. He received intravenous antibiotics of every description with little effect. He'd had so many different antibiotics administered to him during his admissions to Valleyview, this new infection resisted treatment. While the nurses debrided the wound regularly, it became evident he would need plastic surgery. As his flesh sloughed off, the tendons of his lower leg became visible. If the infected wound became worse, he could lose his leg.

Ogden, being a small local hospital, couldn't offer the specialized surgery Ron required so he was transferred to Valleyview Hospital again for preoperative care and following that, plastic surgery.

After Ron's surgery, I made an appointment to see Doctor Fraser, Ron's plastic surgeon. At two o'clock sharp on a blustery February afternoon, I walked into his office. He peered across his desk through thick black-rimmed spectacles and greeted me with a wide smile.

"Your son's surgery turned out well but I'm concerned about his after care. I'm aware of his living situation and his continued use of drugs. Of course, that's a major concern for us as it must be for you but before his release from hospital, I'd like you and Ron to see the social worker and look into securing a suitable housing placement for him. He'll need his dressings changed on a regular basis by a home care nurse and that would be impossible in his present situation. I'll forward my notes on to the social worker."

There were many people in the medical profession I thought of as angels of mercy. This skilled yet unassuming man had to be numbered among them. I followed his instructions and set up an appointment with Clara Meadows, the Valleyview Hospital social worker overseeing Ron's case.

I found Clara's tiny office on the fourth floor. When I entered the room, her files, piled one on top of the other on the desk, hid her assistant's ample figure. I closed the door behind me and stuffed myself into the only other chair in the office. Every available wall space held either sticky notes or a memo board with papers pinned on it in a haphazard fashion.

"Hi, I'm Cindy," the assistant greeted me. "Clara had to go down to the third floor. She'll be back in a minute. Let me see…Ronald Evans. Yes, I've got his file right here."

I couldn't imagine how she could find Ron's file in all that mess but there it sat, as if by magic, on the desk in front of her. The door opened, hitting the back of my chair and a tall dark woman squeezed past me to pick up the file.

"Mrs. Evans, I'm Clara Meadows. Please excuse the mess. Poor Cindy has to put up with this all day. At least I can get out of here and visit clients. Now let's see what we can do about Ron."

"Doctor Fraser told me you might be able to find a placement for him," I told her. "He told me Ron will need home care after he leaves the hospital. He's been living on the street."

"I know, Mrs. Evans. I've been trying to locate something for him. It's difficult though. For one thing, the places I've contacted so far don't have wheelchair access. Those that do won't consider him because of his drug use. He's one of those difficult-to-place clients but while he's in Valleyview, I'll keep on trying to find something. Just leave it with me."

"I know Ron's involved with drugs, mainly marijuana. It seems to help his nerve pain. But he's a good person at heart. He isn't a danger to anyone."

"It's not Ron we're concerned about, Mrs. Evans. It's the drug culture itself. Any group home we find for Ron must protect the other clients in their care. They can't have them exposed to the criminal element."

I noticed Cindy lower her head and thought, *she's familiar with the system and she doesn't look too hopeful.* I left Clara's office not certain they would be able to find Ron a home.

"I'm so tired, Mom," he cried one day. "I know I can't live on my own. I can't live with you and Dad, but I can't live on the street either. Mom, I need help." After so long a time of being sick and tired at last Ron had begun to realize that alcohol and drugs might not be the answer to his problems.

His last three words gave me a glimmer of hope. We spoke with the social worker at the hospital once more and after talking to Ron she arranged for him to attend drug and alcohol counselling as an inpatient. Following his discharge from hospital, he spent additional time at their drug and alcohol addictions clinic. Upon his discharge from the clinic, the outpatient services in the community took over.

The wait for a long-term recovery bed began. Jeff and I allowed him to bunk with us in a small corner of the house as long as he remained drug and alcohol free so his home care nurse felt comfortable when she visited to change Ron's dressings.

"One slip, Ron…, " Jeff warned, "one little slip and you're out of here. Is that understood?"

"Yeah, Dad. I hear you loud and clear."

In the meantime I did some research on the internet and learned there were some excellent drug and alcohol rehabilitation programs available. The only catch was they were not available to him. Most rehabilitation facilities made no provision for wheelchair clients. I found only one long-term addiction facility in the area that accepted wheelchair clients. They had one wheelchair accessible room and that was already occupied.

"I think I'd like to try living on my own again, Dad. I hate to say this, but you and Mom are getting kind of old to be looking after me."

"Ha! I could take you on any day, old buddy," Jeff drawled.

"No. I think he's right, Jeff," I said, agreeing with Ron. "I'm exhausted running around doing everything for you two."

The mood in the house had changed once more. Jeff and I had let down our guard somewhat but when Kevin came in for a visit, he wouldn't let his little brother off the hook so easily.

"He's not going to stop his drug habit overnight, you know. So don't you two get your hopes up or it'll all come crashing down on you again. If he wants to try living on his own, then it'll have to be under some pretty strict rules. I know all about his medical issues but I wouldn't trust that guy as far as I could throw him when it comes to drugs."

After months of waiting for the non-existent rehabilitation bed, Ron decided to forget that route and instead, continue seeing his community counsellor. Between that and his attendance at regular AA and NA meetings, it seemed enough to keep him on track. He had kept his word and stayed away from his old acquaintances. He became determined to attend every meeting possible. Through the support of his Alcoholics Anonymous and Narcotics Anonymous groups, he fought his battle with addiction. On some occasions, one of his AA pals would give him a lift to and from meetings but most often he used the Transit Bus equipped for wheelchairs to get around town. It seemed to Jeff and me that he'd begun to assert his independence once again.

We knew his stay with us could not be permanent. We had crowded together in our little house and no one had any real privacy. We contacted our local health unit for assistance and the social worker at the Ogden office agreed Ron's precarious health prevented him from living on his own. Again, the lineup for suitable accommodation for the adult handicapped remained over a year long. With Ron's history of drug addiction, we realized the prospect of finding a government-sponsored placement for him looked grim.

One day the housing coordinator suggested that we consider a private boarding house facility nearby. Ron happened to be in the hospital again, so Jeff and I went to look at the house. Most of the clients were independent to a degree and all could come and go as they pleased. They cleaned their own rooms and while we were there, we noticed one fellow doing his laundry. One of the women in residence helped serve the meals. All of the clients suffered from one disability or another. It proved to be a "mixed bag". All of the residents had been deemed, as had Ron, difficult to place but the room he would occupy appeared large enough, so he would be able to wheel around comfortably. When Jeff and I next visited him at the hospital, we told him about the house and he agreed to give it a try. I felt relieved. At least I knew he'd have company, a warm bed to sleep in at night and three meals a day.

At Valleyview Hospital, before he got into the transfer ambulance, he confessed, "I'm scared, Mom. Drugs are everywhere. When I'm in pain it's hard to deal with the temptation to take drugs but I'll try, Mom. This time I promise, I'll really try."

EPILOGUE

Ron's health has improved. Although not the life any of us envisioned for him, he is accepting of his new circumstances. His fellow residents have become his other family. He will forever be dependent upon his wheelchair and may not marry or be blessed with children of his own. The excruciating nerve pain in his leg remains his constant companion. His acquired brain injury, without doubt, remains a serious roadblock to his independence, and future goals. He continues to battle the recurrent infections contracted during his time on the street. He lives in fear he may slip again and be dragged down into the oblivion of drug addiction.

Those of us who know and love him still hold on to the hope of a brighter future for him. We hope that one day he will find within himself the confidence and strength he needs to live by his childhood declaration of independence: "Let go! I can do it by myself."

I try to let him go. I struggle to heed the warnings, the words of wisdom from loving family members and concerned professionals. I still recall the day Jeff said, "We have to let him go." He had pointed out the obvious. "You can't fix it."

Today, when I look around at photos of our family, I pause. My gaze falls upon pictures of Ron. In one I see a chubby infant, full of life and gurgling with laughter. In another, I glimpse my seven-year-old, posing with pride in his soccer uniform. I feel laughter in my heart when I look at one of him as a goofy adolescent, mugging in front of the camera alongside his buddies. In the last, I discover a young man, full of hope, eyes focused on the future, all decked out in his first tailored suit, never to be worn again except at weddings and funerals because it isn't "cool".

As Jeff once said, "Ron's in there somewhere, Jan. We just have to find a way to reach him." Although I've come to accept the fact of Ron's disabilities, I don't believe I'll ever be able to let go – to let go of the memory of the boy I once knew. Every now and then when I'm with him, I hear him laugh in a certain way, or make a particular gesture and he's with me once more. For a brief moment, I see the boy he used to be – the man he could become and I have hope.

Ron is in there somewhere.

14020529R00107

Made in the USA
Charleston, SC
15 August 2012